"It is an experiential immersion in the preverbal, in the atmospheres, temperatures, rhythms, and the bodily equivalents not recognised as such, but as they are experienced in a shared return [...] The authors' writings introduce us into the experience of their inner laboratories, making us appreciate their atmospheres, rhythms, and styles, and the astuteness and elegance of their research. The illustrative, essential and illuminating clinical parts depict the various stories and situations with the trusty brushstrokes of the expert analyst, and provide the reader with numerous sensations of surprise at the depth of understanding they are able to instil."

From the Foreword by **Stefano Bolognini**,
Past President of the Italian Psychoanalytic Society,
Past President of the International Psychoanalytic Association,
Chair of the IPA Inter-Regional Encyclopedic
Dictionary of Psychoanalysis

W0018407

Extending the Psychoanalytic Listening Paradigm

Extending the Psychoanalytic Listening Paradigm: Listening with all the Senses guides readers through the nuances of non-verbal communication in the analytic setting.

Presenting a dialogue between three eminent psychoanalysts, this book is made up of numerous case studies and commentaries on patients presenting difficulties with symbolisation, including borderline and primitive mental states. Each analyst presents a different aspect of psychoanalytic listening – body, action, and speech – from a different perspective, before the three come together to analyse these situations. The authors highlight the importance of listening as a device for the analyst, showing how it is used not only to make the repressed emerge, to repair what is traumatic and to activate the continuity of the self, but also as a contribution to constructing the subject throughout the sequence of interactions with the other-than-self. The authors propose an extension of the concept of the unconscious and of the tools used by the analyst in the consulting room: the unconscious states not yet verbalised of the first experiences of psychic life are reached through listening to communications that use other sensory communication channels outside of the verbal.

Bookended by a preface from Stefano Bolognini and an afterword from Francesco Barale, this accessible yet thorough volume is a vital tool for any psychoanalyst or psychotherapist.

Tiziana Bastianini is a psychologist, psychoanalyst, and Training and Supervising analyst for the Italian Psychoanalytic Society and IPA. She has worked with young adults in a mental health service, and previously worked in psychiatric clinics. She lives and works in Rome, Italy.

Anna Ferruta is a psychologist, psychoanalyst and Training and Supervising analyst for the Italian Psychoanalytic Society and IPA. She is a member of the editorial board of the *International Journal of Psychoanalysis*. She specialises in serious diseases and primitive mental functioning, and is a consultant and supervisor in psychiatric institutions and research centres. She lives and works in Milan, Italy.

Benedetta Guerrini Degl'Innocenti is a psychiatrist, psychoanalyst and Training and Supervising analyst for the Italian Psychoanalytic Society and IPA. She is a member of the editorial board of the *International Journal of Psychoanalysis*. Her areas of interest and research are psychoanalytic work with unrepresented mental states, transgenerational issues related to the body and the transmission of psychoanalysis. She lives and works in Florence, Italy.

Extending the Psychoanalytic Listening Paradigm

Listening with all the Senses

Tiziana Bastianini, Anna Ferruta and
Benedetta Guerrini Degl'Innocenti

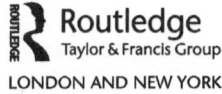

Routledge
Taylor & Francis Group

LONDON AND NEW YORK

Designed cover image: Stone #3 2023, Oil on Canvas (50x70 cm)
© Marta Dell'Angelo *Courtesy of the Artist*

First English edition published 2025
by Routledge
4 Park Square, Milton Park, Abingdon, Oxon, OX14 4RN

and by Routledge
605 Third Avenue, New York, NY 10158

Routledge is an imprint of the Taylor & Francis Group, an informa business

First Italian edition published by Giovanni Fioriti Editore, Rome, 2021
First English edition published by Routledge 2025
The English translation rights arranged through Rightol Media
Email: copyright@rightol.com

ISBN: 978-1-032-89798-1 (hbk)
ISBN: 978-1-032-80220-6 (pbk)
ISBN: 978-1-003-54464-7 (ebk)

DOI: 10.4324/9781003544647

Typeset in Times New Roman
by codeMantra

Contents

Foreword   ix
STEFANO BOLOGNINI

1   **"Psychic intensities": Listening to heterogeneous ways in
    which the unconscious emerges**   1
    TIZIANA BASTIANINI

    *"Listening with all the senses": Metapsychologically widening
        the paradigm of psychoanalytic listening 1*
    Catching the currents of the unconscious 9
    *Brief reflections on the theme of symbolisation: At the origin of
        the non-represented 12*
    *Listening to the negative: Implications of the analytic pair for the
        psychic economy 15*
    *Listening to forms of unconscious intersubjective
        construction 20*
    Semiotic gestures: "The murmur of things" 22
    A fundamental question: "Investigating the caesura" 23
    *Listening to excess: "That nothing, that too much." A different
        reflection on the dimensions of the traumatic 28*
    The body knows: Brief clinical reflections 31
    *Listening to "the blue note": Reflections on the COVID-19
        period 36*
    References 42

2   **Embodied unconsciouses: In the beginning was action**   47
    BENEDETTA GUERRINI DEGL'INNOCENTI

    Daniel and the edge of chaos 49
    *The day after: Looking himself in the face so as not to lose
        himself 50*
    Giving form to the object 52

*Analytic device and symbolic transformation: Giving form to the
    formless 55*
*Giving psychic form to the beginnings of experience: From
    action to representation 56*
In the beginning was action 57
*The work of the psyche-soma: From intercorporeality to
    communication in speech 59*
Giulia: A powerful and irresistible drive to represent 61
To conclude 64
References 66

3   Openings for listening to words   69
ANNA FERRUTA

Overture – a clearing in the forest of symbols 69
Absolute listening "not greedy" for meanings 71
The sonic material of island-words 73
The forms of presence of the object that listens 75
Intensities of the word 78
Condensation of the word 80
Power of the "magic" word 82
The word as a way out of the subject's "enigmatic privacy" 88
Listening to silence 88
An envelope of words: the psychic skin 93
Immersed in a bath of words 97
References 100

**Afterword: On some aspects of contemporary psychoanalysis:
beyond interpretation?**   103
FRANCESCO BARALE

Transference 104
The device and the setting 108
*Symbolisation and the "symbolising function"
    of the object 109*
Factors of transformation (cure) 110
Intrapsychic and interpsychic 112
Problems and questions 113
References 117

Index   *121*

Foreword

Stefano Bolognini

Readers of psychoanalysis at the present time may experience a sense of intercultural vastness that is wonderfully stimulating and at the same time subtly disturbing, or even a cause of anxiety: so many things, so many observations, so many thoughts, and an infinite number of new perspectives and fields, which open the mind and introduce new scenarios and unexpected connections, but may also disorientate by the frightening complexity of their codes, contents, and even methods.

Everything changes, everything is evolving, we know that well enough; and, for those who have been inhabiting specialist territory for many years, how far-off seem the times when the fundamental paradigms described by the pioneers of psychoanalysis were overall quite simple, homogeneous, capable of being summed up in formulae which imprinted themselves enduringly in our minds and guaranteed that our initial idea of psychoanalysis was strongly, almost universally representative!

The typical patient four or five decades ago was still the neurotic. From a psychoanalytic viewpoint, the psychotic was what lay beyond the Pillars of Hercules, something that a few courageous souls ventured to study and treat. The borderline was a bizarre object that was beginning to be spoken about as an occasional but scarcely manageable variant. The narcissistic personality was coming into view on the horizon as something still rather indistinct and understood in highly diverse ways by its various authors; and amid the complexity the categorising diagnostic schemata were held in high regard for the reassuring guidance they gave. Of course, this guidance was quite often thrown off course by the reality of the clinical encounter, but back then it provided a close enough match, being presented with patients who were more clearly characterised (or even sometimes stereotyped) than they are today.

The main contest, still in play in the early 1970s, was between Freud's first and second models, plus the great innovation of the then "new ways in psychoanalysis" introduced by Klein, which provoked contradictory reactions in analysts, from total adherence to an equally absolute rejection. This mostly depended on the cultural and professional communities in which the analyst had been trained and on analysts' transference to authors who to a large extent replicated profound experiences relating to their parental figures and their later equivalents (Bolognini 2019).

Then the psychoanalytic world became gradually populated by a countless variety of contacts, exchanges, and openings onto the new, thanks to the translation of articles and books, attendance at conferences, national and international meetings, wider direct knowledge of the English language, and finally access to the internet with seminars, debates, webinars, and working groups. The ritual celebration of certain formulae, both in sessions and in shared theoretical and clinical reflection, has been replaced with increasing rapidity by new joint visions, by cross-fertilisation not only between different psychoanalytic schools but also between different disciplines.

Psychoanalysis has encountered the neurosciences, sociology, studies of perinatal infancy, the science of group and community organisation, related branches of philosophy, literature and the arts, in a different manner from the past: that is, with the unexpected awareness of a mutual potential advantage, but at the far from negligible cost for us analysts of losing or diminishing a sense of aristocratic uniqueness which had become the basis for a subterranean, self-confirming narcissistic wellbeing that was in fact highly self-centred.

Hence the flourishing over the past 20 years, though not without disputes, of a growing number of interdisciplinary initiatives with experts and scientists in other areas which, on the one hand, have made life more complicated, introducing new concepts and new fields to explore; but, on the other hand, they have enriched us, led us into deeper reflections and reconsiderations about the nature of the things we are concerned with, and have little by little produced modifications that are increasingly evident even in our daily clinical practice.

We have also been led to these new openings by our practice, by the need to work with patients who present with forms of pathology and ways of being and relating that are very different from those of the past.

I won't go into a further description of these epochal changes, which I have dealt with at length in a previous paper ("New Forms of Psychopathology in a Changing World: A Challenge for Psychoanalysis in the Twenty-First Century." *The Italian Psychoanalytic Annual*, 2020) which reprised and updated Gaddini's study from 40 years earlier but, on the back of that, will simply pose a holding question: have we increased the quantity of our scientific exchanges with other disciplines, and consequently widened our analytic vision, because we have benefited from the new possibilities for connection and are eager to share in other people's interesting attainments, or are we instead engaging with them in order to patch up a theoretical and conceptual apparatus that was struggling to address the substantial changes in pathologies and in humanity's ways of being and relating?

I leave it to everyone else to establish which is the chicken and which is the egg, and point out that these thoughts are closely connected to the frontline position occupied by this volume, which from the outset introduces the reader to innovative territories of psychoanalytic investigation: the attention being given by many contemporary analysts to what has not been represented and integrated in the mind in a physiological way and instead stays in the individual, waiting to be recovered, shared with someone, represented, transformed, and reintegrated in a liveable and usable form.

As a result psychoanalysis is becoming ever more a discipline that is in fact confronted by, and immersed in, sensory psycho-corporeal experientiality, co-experienced and shared within the analytic couple, as much as a technique which classically tends to lead the patient towards the processes of symbolisation, with interpretative activities that to some extent require more highly developed functions than those available to many patients who are seeking psychoanalysis today.

It is an experiential immersion in the preverbal, in the atmospheres, temperatures, rhythms, and the bodily equivalents not recognised as such, but as they are experienced in a shared return that seems intrinsically to recall the scholastic "peripatetic axiom" cited by Thomas Aquinas in *De Veritate*: "*Nihil est in intellectu quod non sit prius in sensu,*" and endorses an initial psycho-corporeal basis for what can be mentalised and integrated if the developmental vicissitudes are able to evolve in an appropriate manner; or vice versa, what can be cared for and healed if traumas, deficits, or various obstructive causes prevent mental integration.

Exploring this huge field is a difficult task and culturally and scientifically highly risky, so it is appropriate here for me to share with the reader some elements of knowledge about who is addressing it in this volume. I will say straight away that the three authors are "frontline" psychoanalysts, part of the advance guard.

All three are at the forefront of scientific activity in Italian and international psychoanalysis, both in terms of their own contributions in papers, books, and presentations at conferences, and their administrative roles in their respective institutional settings. They are cutting-edge practitioners, committed to theoretical and clinical dialogue with Italian and foreign colleagues, acknowledged at the highest levels for the quality of what they bring.

But something else unites them besides their shared individual excellence: all three are interested in the new, in what is emerging, whatever opens new doors to psychoanalytic understanding beyond what is already consolidated in our field of research.

In a certain sense all three are acutely sensitive and perceptive about movements in this area, picking up the signals of what promises to be useful, or already is, whatever may potentially be fertile in the sphere of clinical psychoanalytic treatment: in other words, whatever is in fact modifying our profession but still needs to be thought about and formulated more explicitly and widely in order to become genuinely common property.

But here we reconnect to the theme of the difficult growing complexity of current psychoanalysis, the theme with which I began my introduction to this exciting volume: the work of recognising these new theoretical and clinical visions and the wholesale reorganisation they entail is not, and cannot be, simple or easy.

Whoever attempts and achieves this must have an uncommon capacity (in the literal sense, as in physics) for theoretical knowledge: a special liveliness and also, I would say, a nose for interdisciplinary contributions from various sources, selecting them from the myriad offers in circulation; a fluid and precise associative function which enables them to create appropriate, and not approximate, connections between the usable elements that are collected; and then to "work" the dough that is being composed in such a way that those elements aren't merely juxtaposed one on top of the other, but come to create a picture, a whole view, of an observable "object" which can be experienced, comprehended, and endowed with sense for whoever comes into contact with it. To sum up, anyone who takes on such an ambitious and complex task must first of all be up to the job, and must also be sustained by a substantial basic confidence in the possibility of creating an area of interest and shared play with the reader.

Our three authors have these capacities.

Their writings introduce us into the experience of their inner laboratories, making us appreciate their atmospheres, rhythms, and styles, and the astuteness and elegance of their research.

The illustrative, essential and illuminating clinical parts depict the various stories and situations with the trusty brushstrokes of the expert analyst, and provide the reader with numerous sensations of surprise at the depth of understanding they are able to instil. At the same time, however, they always frankly point out how such important therapeutic advances and clarifications, recounted for the sake of brevity in very sober case studies, are in fact the product of years of work with each patient. For example, they cite cases where an apparently banal phrase "dropped in" by the patient at the start of treatment acquires a substantial and fully comprehensible sense only after a long elaboration together in the sessions.

If we are to acknowledge in an integrated way the value and usefulness of theoretical and clinical openness to the new in psychoanalysis, whether this refers to interdisciplinary acquisitions or to explorations in areas that are still poorly mapped (such as the preverbal, the pre-subjective, the interaction and equivalences between the psychic and the corporeally pre-representational), we need gratitude to and recognition of the Masters who have gone before, studying their work in depth, not with a religious attitude or defensively idealising them.

We need to have internalised and truly introjected the essence of interest and research in the most authentic analytic spirit. It is also necessary to maintain a strong curiosity about what we know we don't know, as well as what we don't know we do know; and curiosity about the new, what is waiting to be known, felt, thought, connected, integrated, and acquired in the person and the professional role of a psychoanalyst, until it can become usable and shareable with others.

In this small but – I repeat without hesitation – extraordinarily valuable book we find this substance, this high quality of exploration and elaboration.

But I will add a final note: don't limit yourselves to "what" these three authors – each in their own way – have brought together and investigated; also relish "how" they have developed and worked on it.

Catch the quality of the combination between the fluid and wholly natural, seemingly divergent associations (references to theory, clinical practice, literature, mythology, cinema) and their immediate elaboration by the authors, always solidly concentrating on scientific observation and its translation into theory in the service of technique. Maintaining such an integrated and harmonious disposition is always difficult, especially in times of important scientific and cultural change, and requires – among other things – a skilful level of suspension.

   Not everyone has such a refined capacity, and when we encounter it we should give it the recognition and appreciation it deserves as a fortunate opportunity for the reader who these days wanders with understandable uncertainty in the almost infinite plankton of the countless specialist publications in this sector.

References

Bolognini S. (2019). New Forms of Psychopathology in a Changing World: A Challenge for Psychoanalysis in the Twenty-First Century. *The Italian Psychoanalytic Annual*, 2020.
Aquinas T. (n.d.). *De Veritate*, q. 2 a. 3 arg. 19.

Chapter 1

"Psychic intensities"

Listening to heterogeneous ways in which the unconscious emerges

Tiziana Bastianini

"Listening with all the senses": Metapsychologically widening the paradigm of psychoanalytic listening

I wish to start with two quotes, from Freud and from Green, that help to step into the topic I am addressing: "If his lips are silent, he chatters with his finger-tips; betrayal oozes out of him at every pore" (Freud 1901, p. 78). "The analyst does not listen solely with his ears, but with his entire body … Without the dimension of affect, analysis is a vain and sterile enterprise" (Green 1994, p. 313).

Faced with the complexity of contemporary clinical practice, which is infused with multiple flows of subjectivity characterised by unstable, intermittent and fragile equilibria, and by a lability of boundaries, all of which alter its identitary and narcissistic set-ups, psychoanalytic thought is being asked to keep pondering the fundamental postulates of "*the psychoanalytic encounter,*" which means continually asking new questions. "Two people talking in a room" (Nissim Momigliano 1984; Ferruta 2015) *communicate* on different conscious and unconscious levels via numerous channels which first of all need the other, an Other capable of *adopting a listening position*, listening to "affective intensities." These are "psychic forces," sometimes raw affective states, deprived of the possibility of access to ideational and verbal representation, but they still reveal embryonic traces of a psyche *searching for an experience of a communicative link with a "transformative object"* able to adopt a psychic position from which to receive these communications.

This focus, where the evolution of our understanding of different psychic functionings is critically important, has brought renewed attention to the analyst–patient matrix, to the transference–countertransference dialogue. In other words, to the necessity of investigating the forms of "psychic work" required for understanding psychic formations that may be seeking the active involvement of the other in a shared unconscious communication through psychic forms expressed in action (Bastianini 2019); new functions of figuration and representation, specific forms of shared psychic work *à deux*, especially when the reverberation of the traumatic register confronts us with an amalgam of heteromorphic psychic materials that may be reactivated in behaviours, acts and bodily sensations (Roussillon 2018). It is possible that the couple's psychic work and the analyst's work on her

DOI: 10.4324/9781003544647-1

countertransference, which may include unconscious responses in the form of action (enactments), will enable these traumatic materials to make the transition and exist in the register of verbal thought.

It was in any case clear to Freud that language must lead to "understanding" (1895) in a sense that includes the verbal and the non-verbal, and indeed he would later assert that, "'speech' must be understood not merely to mean the expression of thought in words but to include the speech of gesture and every other method ... by which mental activity can be expressed" (Freud 1913, p. 176).

A listening that is organised according to a polyphonic and polysemic principle based on the varied places and forms in which the unconscious reveals itself in the link (Kaës 2015); a listening endowed with a specific "metabolising-transformative" function and which we could provisionally define as the psychoanalyst's *distinctive psychic work*, conceived in the singular intersubjective exchange which can then be expressed in revealing its own *semiotic, metaphorical and symbolic function*.

From this perspective, the conceptualisation of what we could call a metapsychological widening of the paradigm of psychoanalytic listening[1] is concerned with hypotheses that arise from the encounter between the method of conceptualisation and psychoanalytic practice and are defined *through the goals of clinical care and knowledge* in their indivisible correlations and extensions.

More specifically, this kind of conceptualisation requires us to consider a theoretical axis which, based on listening, fans out along a sequence of concepts such as countertransference, reverie, imagination and the analyst's intuitive thinking in the session, considered within a dialogic matrix that characterises the analytic couple's psychic work (Botella and Botella 2001; Bastianini and Ferruta, 2018). In the link and by means of the link, the unconscious gives form to a plurality of expressive configurations directed towards the nearest human being (Freud 1895). In this context *the notion of intersubjective resonance* becomes central, entailing new topographical and economic hypotheses about psychoanalytic listening as a clinical consequence of possible high-intensity exchanges that involve the different transferential phenomenologies and the various associative processes.

In theoretically widening the functions of psychoanalytic listening we have come to consider an *embodied listening* that contemplates the bodily movements and entire self of analyst and patient. This implies extending the concept of associativity; indeed, taking on the psychic in all its extension and multiplicity of codes includes widening the concept of free association or associative thought. It means accepting lines of psychic expression that emerge from a variety of sources, no longer just the verbal world but also a possible expressive sensorimotor associativity linked to sound or image, which sees two or more embodied psychic systems in play and *can be considered an integral and essential part of the analytic set-up. Naturally, this entails considering how the analytic set-up may include the numerous expressive currents of the psychic* (see Bastianini and Ferruta 2018; Bastianini 2019).

So our attention *also* turns to the psychosomatic resonances as unconscious reverberations of the communication between patient and analyst (Jacobs 1991, 2007), capable of revealing specific *qualities and quantities* of the affective investment that is in play. In fact, we know that the bodily movements which accompany the act of listening are the outward sign of unconscious forms of expression that reveal configurations of feeling which run in parallel to the verbal exchange (Bucci 1997; Searles 1979; Stern 2004, 2010). I am thinking especially about the vital dynamic forms of movement "because movement is the dynamic of representation" (Green 2005, p. 19) able to evoke in us the perception of *internal forces capable of making us resonate* with them and endowed with an intrinsic vectorial intentionality as we communicate (Stern 2010).

That is, I am thinking of Nadia Fusini's (2010) *"passionate speech"* made of gestures – i.e. the body – and words, their infinitely repeated reverberations back and forth. Through the dramatisation and staging of what speech cannot yet say, action reveals the potential for a "not-me," a residue of the psychic experience not yet translated or translatable, that will be negotiated in the encounter with another psyche capable of taking on the freight of these communications, transferring them in the direction of a possible symbolisation (Benjamin 2017).

In my opinion, we need to engage with psychic facts in a way that has "as much effect and impact as a physical act can. The range of phenomena communicable in verbal language is extremely poor, limited to the phylogenetically most recent features, those linked to speech" (Riolo 1978; cf. Bastianini 2009a).

We have now been aware for some time that what is grasped with the senses is not a matter of simply transmitting the sensible via the sensory apparatus, and that "even at the periphery, the physiological impression is engaged in relations that were previously considered to be central" (Merleau-Ponty 1945, p. 10). Besides, perception entails a pathic dimension (Bastianini 2009b) that also contains the potential to negativise perception itself.

It is interesting to go back to the Freud of *The Interpretation of the Aphasias* (1891), a study in which he claims that:

> We are still quite ignorant of the elements which contribute to the functional changes that conducted stimuli undergo. We can only presume that the fibre tracts, which reach the cerebral cortex after their passage through other grey masses, have maintained some relationship to the periphery of the body, but no longer reflect a topographically exact image of it. *They contain the body periphery in the same way as... a poem contains the alphabet, i.e. in a completely different arrangement serving other purposes, in manifold associations of the individual elements, whereby some may be represented several times, others not at all.*
>
> (Freud 1891, p. 53, my italics)

From this perspective we observe migrations between psychic agencies, migrations involving the various sources from which we procure our psychic material. They belong to heterogeneous sources that reveal the polysemic complexity of the signs and traces of the processes of being psychically represented, including traces in negative.

In other words, it is necessary to take the affects into account and entrust them with a primary role as a central subjective experience. Their fate may be linked to motor expressions, actions, sensations, conflict, or anxiety as a signal – whatever the case, they will be the vehicle for a message with communicative value, addressed from the outset "towards the nearest human being" (Freud 1892–1899; cf. Bastianini 2019).

So the central question becomes an enquiry into the "analytic probes" necessary for capturing the heart of an experience that advances into psychic territories, the functioning of which reveals a possible impasse in the register of symbolisation and, at the same time, we must take into consideration the multiplicity of communicative registers present in the analytic exchange. From this perspective it becomes equally important to bear in mind Freud's (1912) claim that, if it is properly attuned, the analyst's unconscious is capable of directly capturing what is transmitted by the patient's unconscious. From the same perspective I would also keep in consideration another valuable suggestion by Freud: "everyone possesses in his unconscious mental activity an apparatus which enables him to interpret *other people's reactions*, that is, to undo the distortions which other people have imposed on the expression of their feelings" (Freud 1912–1913, p. 159). The apparatus for interpreting the unconscious of others, in other words, goes hand in hand with the need to maintain the bonds that are indispensable for the subject's biological, affective and relational survival. This is Bowlby's (1969, 1973) territory, the attachment bonds (need for safety) which we tend to think of today as also being a form of affect regulation. After decades of research we know much more about the ways in which the child's identifications appropriate the rules for being and for putting oneself in relation to the other: the unthought known is in fact a form of knowledge that we possess thanks to the earliest experiences of the object world. The sense of what we learn is stored inside us in forms, images, and affective schemata which govern our perspectives, our states of mind (Bollas 2007).

From this perspective it may be helpful to point out that "the subject of sensation," to which this chapter will try and give a different psychoanalytic status, is a subject *with a historical thickness*, in constant and complex dialogue with the present. It is not "a thinker who notices a quality," still less an inert material that could be passively affected or modified by it, but "*a power that is born together with a certain existential milieu or that is synchronized with it*" (Merleau-Ponty 1945, p. 219, my italics). In this view, moreover, there is particular significance in current research on *interbrain synchronisation*[2] and the connected *mirroring* mechanisms in the expression of the gestures and in sensorimotor and verbal communications. On this subject, in his weighty preface to the writings of Ricœur (2020), Barale claims that psychoanalytic experience – inevitably caught "between force and sense" and irreducible to a linguistic reality – is in fact the terminal point "of a very dense thickness of modulations, re-actualisations, transformations, transits, and shifting emotional investments and affects which is the indispensable – in a certain sense 'material' – intersubjective condition whereby new meanings can appear and be recognised" (Ricoeur 2020, p. 12).

So we have to ask ourselves: if we consider two or more embodied psychic systems against a background of the conceptualisation of object–subject in their possible permutations of *presence–absence–recognition* from which arise variously organised qualities of the psychic, do we need a renewed metapsychology of listening? That is to say, the ability to refine our conceptual grids, from which arise new paths of psychoanalytic technique that are translated into broader conceptions of our curative tools. When listening is directed to heterogeneous psychic materials, some of which are situated beyond representation in speech, we have to ask ourselves what type of psychic work is needed by the analyst in order to take on that *quantity of affect* which impacts on her listening and prompts her to make available all her registers of functioning and gathering data – which also include *perceiving, imagining, hallucinating* (Botella and Botella 2001; La Scala 2017; Bastianini 2019) in a renewed exploration into a hypothetical "metapsychology of the analyst's mental processes during analysis" (Ferenczi, 1928, p. 96). When we investigate the heterogeneity of the processes of derivation, transformation, and correlation as the constant flow of countless psychic productions emerges, oscillating from one field to the other of the psyche-soma, we become ever more aware of the complexity of the transformative processes and their possible intelligibility. Therefore, in answer to the previous question, the need to include the characteristics of the mind's psychosensory area (Gaddini 1969) demands a broadening of metapsychology and an awareness that we should pay attention to the cruxes inherent in the gradual reciprocity between formation of the representational functions and the construction of the subject's continuity between bodily expression and expression in language. The psychosensory components are in fact silently but potently active in the analytic couple's unconscious communication and in the configuration of its transitional space. A base function exists, structured on the five senses, capable of giving life to "perceptual experiences" of various kinds which lack verbal language. These are communications founded on sensorimotor gestures, actions, behaviours, and non-verbal expressions, which reveal an affectivity expressed in an "economic-semiotic" mode, testimony to a ceaseless psychic work of transformation and communication. As Bion reminds us:

> When a patient comes to see me, there is, in fact, a body which I can see for myself, and to that extent I can fall back on the evidence of my senses and on the information which my senses bring me. I don't think that we can afford to ignore what our senses tell us, because the facts are very few anyway.
>
> (Bion 2005, pp. 1–2)

At the clinical level this means recognising that sensory, affective, and somatic elements have the potential for meaning and language, the status of precursors to representation (De Toffoli 2009; Matthis 2000). If "every sensation includes a seed of dream" (Merleau-Ponty 1945, p. 223) in which we are immersed, we must in fact be able to suppose a mind structured on the five senses and able to bring various forms of thought to life (cf. Bastianini 2019).

Early on, in *The Interpretation of Dreams*, Freud (1899) speaks about forms of thought inherent in the primary processes and the numerous forms of inscription connected to them: visual, acoustic, tactile and kinaesthetic traces, and perhaps other kinds too, which will only partly make the transition into the ranks of verbal symbolisation, while continuing to innervate the other forms of thought that characterise the unconscious and the formation of dream (Finelli 2017. The transformations that lead from sensory data to verbally expressible thoughts are based on the intuition of unconscious forms with a strong affective valence, experienced as qualities of touch, heat, pressure, sound, light, rhythm and oscillation which can be produced by internal or external perceptions (Bion 1965). We know that sensory stimuli – endogenous and exogenous – determine "nascent movements" enveloped in vital significance (Merleau-Ponty 1945). Before unconscious fantasy can become an imaginative representation – i.e. be dreamed – it is experienced through the body (Boyer 1999; De Toffoli 2009; Gaddini 1981). In other words, there is a sensory contiguity which sets up a primal "relationship of shape to the feeling of enclosure, of beat to the feeling of rhythm, of hardness to the feeling of edgedness" (Ogden 1989, p. 32). Freud believed that the Ego derived from bodily sensations, in the first place those proceeding from the surface of the body (Freud 1927). Therefore, from this perspective the experience of self represents first of all a non-reflective condition, a "sensory coming to be" (Winnicott 1956) derived from the needs of a bodily Ego that only gradually, through the imaginative working-through of physical experience in the mother–child relationship, will become a psychic Ego.

From his viewpoint as a psychoanalyst and researcher into child development, Daniel Stern reminds us that from birth onwards babies are at the centre of sensations, perceptions, actions, cognitions, internal states of motivation and states of consciousness that are not yet self-reflective, and they know them directly in terms of experiences of intensity, forms, temporal schemata, vital affects and pleasurable affects (Stern 1985). These very early modes of experience operate over the whole course of life beneath consciousness as an experiential matrix for all subsequent states of subjectivity.

Moreover, Varela (1991) reminds us that the relationship between living beings and their environments is one of mutual specification and codetermination, a continual evolution of subject and world in a structural coupling that becomes *the product and the trace* of unique histories.

The Ego and its body, with the pleasure connected to it, are the first trace of a "wellbeing of one's own" at the origin of life that is nurtured by the pleasure obtained from the other's caregiving – a pleasure experienced in one's own flesh (Aulagnier 1979). At the centre of the experience there is a body that can move, touch, show itself and form a connection with other bodies; a body that can give and receive pleasure. So there is also an interchange of "subjective" and physical states: right from the earliest sensory experiences, even before a psychic subject has been born, the body in fact has intense investments passing through it. The way the sensory impressions at the origin of life are capable of being bound to emotions through the complex mirroring of somatic signals in relation to affective states constitutes the basis for understanding how emotions will organise the feeling of self. Over time these traces will become symbolic material and a foundation of the reflective function, which will in turn give form to the expression of the subjective idiom (I am alluding to a sense of self at the preverbal beginning, which will act as the basis of all subsequent acquisitions). As Modell reminds us, the vitality of the *private self* depends on the ability to generate meaning: "I propose that the unconscious can be thought of as a neurophysiological process that has the potential to generate meaning" (Modell 1993, p. 144).

Over time we have understood how much "experience" is registered in our bodies. Nature and culture do not constitute separate levels of functioning but are reciprocally "contaminated" in the early periods of development as the neuronal networks are being "sculpted" (Bastianini 2006). We only experience emotions such as anger, joy, distress and sexual desire because we are equipped with a suitable cerebral apparatus for generating such emotions. These emotions in turn generate neurophysiological functionings whose chemistry alters and influences the neural pathways. Our evolution as biological beings has enabled the development of culture and human language which in turn generate metaphors, psychic perspectives, through which we experience our own bodies.

Bearing in mind that, as Gaddini writes, "The mental is based on the organic and … the mental quality of a determined psychic function consists primarily in having a sense that it does not have physiologically" (1981, p. 496). The organic is, to use a different conceptual metaphor suggested by Panksepp (2012), "the ancestral source of our emotional mind."

Gallese (see Ammaniti and Gallese 2014) recalls that the mirror neurone system links speech to movement. When words are uttered they activate the mirror neurones corresponding to the actions and movements being verbally described. From this perspective, words are symbols incarnated in the experience that conveys implicit levels of functioning. Metaphors are not only rhetorical figures of speech but fundamental sensorimotor ways of experiencing the world and conceptualising it by means of non-verbal mental categories (Modell 1993). I find Panksepp's (2012) studies of the Seeking System very interesting from this viewpoint: he distinguishes this system from the other fundamental motive forces of the human mind (sexuality, aggression, attachment, etc.) though it is in constant dialogue with them. In this context, we can hardly fail to bear in mind the nexus with Bion's (1959) K-link or Klein's (1932) epistemophilic instinct.

It is in this dual register, between autopoiesis and dyadic regulation that we may be able to locate the hypothesis of the dyadic expansion of consciousness between the child and the mother, a form of intersubjectivity in a psyche thought of as an open system that self-organises and creates its own states of consciousness which may evolve to become mental states endowed with greater complexity and coherence thanks to cooperation with another self-regulated system.[3] The theoretical matrix at the base of this hypothesis, which concerns both the mother-infant dyad and that of analyst and patient, is Thelen and Smith's (1994) conception of non-linear dynamic systems. Or as Tronick reminds us:

> I believe that the social and emotional exchanges between mother and child (and between all human beings) have the potential to extend the individual state of consciousness, a condition with important consequences from the experiential and developmental viewpoint. The hypothesis of the dyadic expansion of consciousness derives from system theory.
>
> (1998, p. 102)

Naturally, alongside the dyadic expansion of consciousness, we simultaneously find all the psychic work of the subject or the dyad or the wider system of the family group, aimed at the unconscious level at negotiating meanings that will be able to evolve towards symbolic representation or mute areas that will remain in a separate region of the psyche waiting to be expressed one day.

So we are tracking a subject, a living, open psychobiological system in constant dialectic between autopoiesis and epigenesis. Let us, therefore, suppose the existence of a psychic life and forms of thought that are expressed beyond verbal language, or equally that attract into speech traces and inscriptions belonging to sensory dimensions registered in other periods of life (cf. Bion 1962; Fédida 2012; Green 2012; Ogden 2005; Winnicott 1971). How many languages, which concern us as psychoanalysts, can the unconscious speak? A variety of languages that are the origin of psychic expressions which pursue communicative logics different from representation in speech. Put another way, it is a matter of considering "a permanent construction in the formation of the psychic" (Green 2012, p. 116) shot through by a range of defensive processes which should be counterpointed by an analytic listening composed by that infinite psychic work of provisional constructions made from "various psychic materials" (2012, p. 118) which take shape one after the other in the analyst's thought during the session, and which must be able to welcome the force of the emotional turbulences in play. In other words, Anzieu (1996, p. 63) asks us, "Can the logic of verbal thinking take non-verbal logics into account?"

From this perspective, can we hypothesise a listening function that tries to arrive at forms of expression of the psychic at the boundaries of verbal thinking *through work that happens in the analyst's mind and aims to achieve symbolising form, as an attempt to connect heterogenous psychic communications – sometimes even through the "knowing" of her own body?* It is important, therefore, that future research in psychoanalysis continues to explore how the different *forms of communication, including those in shared action,* will make different expressive registers resonate in the analyst's listening, gradually being brought back into the logic of verbal thought. Unexpected "connections and consonances" which make possible new forms of psychic life, of "communicative play" between the unconsciouses (Winnicott 1974).

This is a function of analytic listening that may build bridges, nexuses that set up communication between affective levels and states of the polymorphous psyche, and through such forms of joint psychic work (Freud 1938a) *may be able to re-establish and transform topographical and economic boundaries. A psychic operation that is essential in developing a sort of metalanguage able to make the unconscious speak and open it at last to speech: a speech laden with affects, a living speech capable of creating psychic movement in both patient and analyst* (Green 2005).

In other words:

> We gather the material for our work from a variety of sources – from what is conveyed to us by the information given us by the patient and by his free associations, from what he shows us in his transferences, from what we arrive at by interpreting his dreams and from what he betrays by his slips or parapraxes. All this material helps us to make constructions about what happened to him and has been forgotten as well as about what is happening in him now without his understanding it.
>
> (Freud 1938a, pp. 177–178)

Catching the currents of the unconscious

It was about 20 years ago that the debate surrounding the different ways in which the unconscious emerges became denser and more complex. Since it is especially complex to retrace the various threads that have contributed to the expansion of the conceptualisations behind the different forms of unconscious psychic work, I will try to identify some of the principal theories that have helped us to widen our capacity for clinical comprehension (bearing in mind that we may refer both to the contents of the unconscious and to the thought processes that organise it).

Let us try, on this occasion, to conceptualise how our way of understanding unconscious mental processes has changed over the years. This change has involved a movement from the *centrality of the secondary processes of repression* to the centrality of *what has not yet been formulated* (Freud 1895; Stern 2004), not yet lived, for numerous reasons. On the topic of unconscious mental functioning that is not yet representable or represented, I think it is important to distinguish two questions: on the one hand, the consideration of what has not yet been formulated as *becoming*, a potentiality not yet expressed and linked to the future, without a past that tends towards repetition; and, on the other hand, the inherent feature of unconscious mental functioning as an expression of very early traces, traumatic in character, that tend to repeat without memory and are capable of generating emotional states which are inexpressible on the symbolic and metaphorical level, emotional turbulences that can thus only *"present themselves" in the body, in action or the resonances of enactment* (Guerrini Degli Innocenti 2016; Sapisochin 2013). I understand the aim of this repetition as being to communicate the goal of integrating primary psychic material through the unconscious cooperation of another psyche.

We have tried to retrace and bring into focus an area of unconscious psychic functioning and forms of thought that draw their origin from perceptual-emotional, pre-symbolic, pre-linguistic, pre-representational levels. We have also understood that the unconscious psychic can be experienced in many forms: *for a long time, the theory of secondary repression was the only evidence of unconscious productions*, and this did not allow us to observe other forms of unconscious expression such as unconscious perception, unconscious organisation, unconscious communication (Bollas 2009). We have learned to pay close attention and catch more of what is revealed by a person:

> What about the sequence revealed through the tones of voice a person employs to give emphasis to his or her utterances? What about the way that person uses his or her body (hands, feet and, particularly, facial expression) to indicate a sequence of ideas? ... These lines of expression open up the field of unconscious expression even more widely, thickly and deeply.
>
> (Bollas 2009, pp. 18–19)

(Even so, as far back as his 1915 paper, Freud had revealed an unconscious with a wider range than just the repressed, having in mind the great theme of primary repression.)

The extension of clinical practice has provoked a requirement to take account on the conceptual plane of what happens in the consulting room between two or more embodied psyches. From this perspective, taking on the psychic in its full extent and multiplicity includes a broadening *of the concept of free association* or *associative thought*, so as to welcome lines of psychic expression that emerge from various sources like a vast symphonic movement and belong to the sense-domains of the motoric, the expressive, sound, and image, to which we attribute communicative value. Naturally, all this has its correlation in the forms of listening that the analyst can offer in the varied configurations of unconscious reception, "by these means to catch the drift of the patient's unconscious with his own unconscious" (Freud 1922, p. 239). This analytic listening is a constituent part of that infinite psychic work of temporary constructions made from "various psychic materials" that alternate back and forth as they form in the thought of the analyst in the session, a listening capable of taking on the force of the emotional turbulences in play.

The fact that an ever clearer focus has been brought to the formation of the psychic structures, the indivisibility of the drive–object pairing, substantially determined by the inherited disposition (unconscious psychic life begins *in utero*) and by the logic of parental caregiving, has confronted us with a field of psychic knowledge that is constantly being developed but not mentally represented: "before the small child is capable of topographically significant mental representations (involving secondary repression and preconscious processes) the child already knows the basic essentials of human life" (Bollas 1987). This implicit knowing is, by definition, a knowledge that is not symbolised. It is non-verbal, procedural, and unconscious.

Theories of mind which place emphasis on the importance of the experience of being in a relationship from the earliest moments of life highlight an affective learning that bears the strong imprint of the Freud of *Two Principles of Mental Functioning*. In this respect, the theme of "attention and notation" becomes central *in a new openness to the conceptual binomial of perception-consciousness* with the aim of positing *an unconscious perception* of the other's psychic qualities, by means of which to construct forms of affective auto- and hetero-regulation. This is an emotional experience of self-maintained and preserved as a trace, still unthought but helpful for future comprehensions since it will go towards constructing a first system of affective memory which has for a long time been defined in some bodies of theory as *implicit memory or implicit relational knowledge*. This form of knowledge will nevertheless be reworked as the symbolic-verbal capability is acquired.

So let's posit a psychic life and forms of thought, heterogenous in their processes of derivation, transformation, and correlation, which express themselves from one field of the psyche-soma to the other beyond verbal language, or draw into speech traces and inscriptions belonging to sensory, kinetic, and sensorimotor dimensions in other periods of life (cf. Fédida, Ogden, Green). Should we be able to postulate forms of thought without language? We wondered earlier how many languages can be spoken by the unconscious with which we as psychoanalysts are concerned. – various languages which give rise to expressions of the psychic that pursue logics different from representation in words. Put another way, it is a matter of "a permanent construction in the formation of the psychic" (Green 2012):

> the dream-work is not simply more careless, more irrational, more forgetful and more incomplete than waking thought; it is completely different from it qualitatively and for that reason not immediately comparable with it. It does not think, calculate or judge in any way at all; it restricts itself to giving things a new form. (Freud 1899, p. 507)

In other words, we find ourselves faced with a vast territory composed by "the complexity of the processes of the mind" (Freud 1938a, p. 196), conscious and unconscious, determined by the plurality of the traces and temporalities registered in them; past and future, what happened and was never signified by the psyche, but also what never happened and could only take shape as a negative trace. It is in this crucible that we can actualise heterogeneous forms of expression of the psychic, able to convey communications at a high level of affective intensity which are capable of making the psyche of the analyst resonate in the here and now of the present analytic relationship in a specific "work as a double." "This way of working as a double thus operates between two psyches. One of them, demonstrating a remarkable degree of momentary plasticity, reflects what is only potential in the other." In the work of two embodied psychic systems it becomes, "a complex act involving both passiveness and appropriation, revealing and even creating psychic data" (Botella and Botella 2001, p. 84).

> The patient produces before us with plastic clarity an important part of his life-story, of which he would otherwise have probably given us only an insufficient account. He acts it before us, as it were, instead of reporting it to us.
> (Freud 1938a, pp. 175–176)

For Freud, therefore, it is not a matter of remembering the past but of a force acting in the present. So it is no accident that he used the term "*agieren*," taken from the language of the theatre, to indicate not simple evacuative action (acting-out), but the irreducible urge to representation by means of a dramatic act situated in a "theatrical" space.

In *Remembering, Repeating, and Working-Through*, Freud distinguished between two forms of memory: repetition in behaviour and affect (reproduction in action) and symbolic representational memory (reproduction in the psychic field), and emphasised that "making them conscious to the patient" (Freud 1914a, p. 147) could often not be achieved through childhood memories but only by means of the transference which was, in this respect, equivalent to memory. This distinction was the antecedent of the great debate that has absorbed the psychoanalytic community around the topic of therapeutic action. For Freud, repetition in action predominantly concerned repressed psychic contents, but in the same paper, referring to the multiplicity of mnemic forms of what had been forgotten, he also took non-repressed psychic contents into account, "new and deeper-lying instinctual impulses" (Freud 1914a, p. 153) which might have been recorded but, having been rejected, they have only been able to leave a trace in the Id.

To sum up, we should be able to construct a *polysemy, a "polytopia" of the unconscious*, since we need to extend the forms of representation of the psychic along a continuum that runs from the thing to the word and vice versa, from the sensorimotor to the symbol. Put another way, we need to unearth relations of compatibility between the orders of the symbolic and the affective, recalling that language "can only work on material already worked on" (Green 1983).

Brief reflections on the theme of symbolisation: At the origin of the non-represented

In clinical work with borderline states (Green 2012; Roussillon 2006) the question of symbolisation stimulates us to challenge ourselves once again on the theme of absence, loss, separation. In the psychoanalytic tradition, we have often regarded the processes of symbolisation as referring to quite highly developed forms of the capacity to tolerate absence and separateness. In reality we should posit the presence of a primary symbolisation (Anzieu 1985) which unfolds in the presence of the object against a background of capacities embodied by the mother. Indeed, it is in the maternal mind that this capacity takes shape, the ability to put together signals which belong to different registers of psychophysical functioning. There is a profound difference between contemplating the borderline, the lack, transitioning from an experience of psychically borne impotence to a "non-breast" capable of producing thought, and the agonising conditions of traumatic impotence against which the psyche will struggle without being able to produce symbolic solutions. We are further stimulated to journey back into the theme of "the role of illusion in symbol formation" and the effects of the premature loss of faith in the reality created by the Self (Milner 1955).

Winnicott's thinking (1945, 1948) – about how a good enough mother *allows the child to unify its predisposition to hallucinate a pleasant and satisfying encounter* in relation to the first sensations of being immersed in a dependable environment – enables us also to comprehend how the oscillation between the illusion of union and reality of contact with a limiting not-me, *creator of a boundary and a temporality*, may describe the discovery of something new emerging between I and you. From this perspective Winnicott can bring the pairing of primary creativity and perception, the found and the created, into dialogue within the construction of the "transitional object" which has as its referent "symbolism in time." All of this is necessary to describe the long psychic journey which enables the infant to "go towards the object," the journey that is the sign of progress towards lived experience (Winnicott 1971).

> The infant can employ a transitional object when the internal object is alive and real and good enough (not too persecutory). *But this internal object depends for its qualities on the existence and aliveness and behaviour of the external object. Failure of the latter in some essential function indirectly leads to deadness or to a persecutory quality of the internal object.* After a persistence of inadequacy of the external object the internal object fails to have meaning to the infant, and then, and then only, does the transitional object become meaningless too.
>
> (Winnicott 1971, pp. 9–10, my italics)

Naturally, we are aware that, in every human experience, alongside the "good encounter," there may always appear the encounter that opens the way to disappointment, to the bad object and to the bad, frustrating self. If these latter experiences are well moderated and contained in the potential space, within the limits that the child's mind can tolerate, they will create in the subject a *basic faith in the bond and in the reparative potential for resolving and working through conflict, a condition that will give rise to a logic of hope* as an engine of psychic life.

In other words, I would like to try to explore and understand unconscious solutions that structure psychic development on the preverbal, pre-symbolic level: a primary psychic process, a psychic agglomeration of affects, impressions, sensations and drives that, from the beginning, testify to *the event and the psyche's attempts to assimilate it, the intimate correlation between the historical and psychic dimensions*. In the final hypotheses of his theoretical journey, Freud refers to the integration or non-integration of overwhelming experiences that tend to repeat themselves in search of a possible integration; so, at the very end of his life, Freud placed the question of integration at the foundation of Ego-structuring: the Ego can alter itself so as not to succumb. The focus on such expressions of the psychic from a psychoanalytic viewpoint presupposes that our listening undertakes to extend itself *towards plural forms of associativity*, towards a polymorphism of the communicative expressions in which configurations deriving from the different perceptual and sensorimotor forms may run alongside the verbal traces. This results in an amalgam of polymorphous psychic materials mixing together acts, gestures, and bodily sensations in dialogue using figures that are different from verbal representation.

We have previously noted how the affective and emotional communication between patient and analyst happens along numerous pathways, not only those of language (and we have recognised a multiplicity of communicative vectors in language). Another feature that helps us to make hypotheses about such widenings, as we noted earlier, derives from the concept of implicit relational knowledge (Lyons-Ruth 1998, 2003). Implicit knowing is not limited to the universe of non-verbal communication, movements or bodily sensations; it also refers to the affects and the paralinguistic elements of verbal language. Implicit knowing is unconscious in a topographical sense, but it is not dynamically repressed. This opens up some questions about the theme of unconscious perception, a field of knowledge in continuous development but not mentally represented. Before it can construct *topographically significant mental representations* which entail secondary repression and the preconscious processes, *the child already knows the logics of being and of putting oneself in a relationship* (Bollas 1987). This knowledge is a knowing that is not symbolised: that is, it is a matter not of verbal but procedural and unconscious knowledge (in the sense that it is not reflectively conscious).

In this research context, I think it is important to go back and take a wider metapsychological look at the concept of the "economic factor." In other words, I believe it is important to consider an economy of affect that may be located at various levels of symbolisation, from that of genuine linguistic symbolisation to that of affect in action, which may be revealed in behaviour or in the expressions of the body: levels and gradients of symbolisation with which we come into contact within the perspective of the analytic relationship. If "the unconscious ... *was the infantile; it was that part of the self which had become separated off from it in infancy, which had not shared the later stages of its development*" (Freud 1909, p. 177), what must be emphasised is that for Freud the traces of what has passed and been experienced continue to exist affectively and to act in the adult: they are those aspects *which could not be integrated in the development of the individual.* The affective reactions to trauma create an intolerable psychic state that threatens to disorganise and destroy the psychic functions (see Draft K from 1 January 1896 in the correspondence with Fliess). A closer look at the dynamic conception of the nature of trauma highlights the responses that the psychic apparatus is called upon to make use of, the defences that it is in a position to produce: conceptual elaborations that seem to prefigure theoretical developments and subsequent research into *the split-off and/or dissociated aspects of the self.* That which the psyche continues to fear and which destroys its life has already happened, Winnicott reminds us. It is a fact that is maintained hidden in the unconscious:

The unconscious here is *not exactly the repressed unconscious of psychoneurosis,* nor is it the unconscious of Freud's formulation of the part of the psyche that is very close to neurophysiological functioning ... In this special context the unconscious means that *the ego integration is not able to encompass something.*

The ego is too immature to gather all the phenomena into the area of personal omnipotence … The original experience of primitive agony cannot get into the past tense *unless the ego can first gather it into its own present time experience and into omnipotent control now (assuming the auxiliary ego-supporting function of the mother (analyst))*.

(Winnicott 1974, pp. 104–105, my italics)

I am thinking of the girl recalled by Winnicott in *Playing and Reality* who, while she played the other children's games, was always busy daydreaming and as an adult in analysis wanted to bring dreams but could only bring a nighttime fantasy disguised as a dream.

To some extent fantasying has remained static over the whole of this patient's life, that is to say, dating from very early years, the pattern being established by the time that she was two or three. It was in evidence at an even earlier date.

(Winnicott 1971, p. 26)

Winnicott thus connects the origin of "fantasying" to a pre-representational phase and an interference in the transitional space.

In the encounter with a contemporary clinical practice characterised by psychopathological configurations at the root of which we trace significant fissures in the narcissistic disposition, in the feeling of self, we are more and more called upon to engage with complex forms of listening. Today many forms of malaise are expressed across uncertain boundaries, from a viewpoint that is both corporeal and psychic: that is, through "thin-skinned" psychic envelopes – a skin that makes such patients vulnerable to narcissistic wounds, exposed to humiliating feelings of shame. Moreover, we observe in these patients an absolute dependency on their objects and a simultaneous phobic avoidance of them; confusion and scant differentiation in their erotic dynamics; a mixing of pleasant and painful experiences; the pervasive sensation of not living their own lives, or living them as if observing themselves from outside. All these features seem to be organising signs of psychic dynamics that reveal a specific fracture in the area of the symbolising processes and determine expressions of the psychic through heterogeneous modalities. From another perspective we should certainly ask ourselves what kinds of *Kulturarbeit* are proclaimed by such signs of the psychic in the forms of contemporary malaise. What unconscious pacts do they correspond to in the context of the human exchanges between the sexes and the generations? Such a reflection, though fundamental, is beyond the scope of this study.

Listening to the negative: Implications of the analytic pair for the psychic economy

From this research perspective, *interrogating the traumatic factor once again*, we have witnessed a resumption of the dialectical debate about "aspects of the negative": a negative to be explored further in all its potential, from the most physiological negative capability (Bion 1993) originating in the birth of new openings to sense, to the permutations of a negation (Freud 1925a) that triggers the birth of distinctive forms of psychic reality. I am thinking of late Freud and the areas of research that were initiated around the themes of denial, rejection, and abolition, understood as "primary defence mechanisms." The negative takes shape between the psychic dimensions of absence, loss, and void, running all the way to negative hallucination. Such forms of psychic functioning that reveal "traumatic" traces, are translated into anxieties and disturbances of the processes of subjectivation and symbolisation.

Lastly, from this perspective, we wonder *how are the traces of the negative revealed in analytic listening.*

When, in the transference, a patient reveals defensive modes characterised by functionings involving the work of the negative such as denial, negation, affective disinvestment, and negative hallucination, they reveal a relationship with the internal and external objects characterised by the splitting-dissociation (Ferenczi, 1928) that is helpful in confronting a potential psychic disorganisation. We posit a fundamental difference between what has been deleted, subjected to a negative hallucination (Green 2011), and what has instead been repressed: that is, "noted" and subsequently forgotten. We are faced with a form of negativisation closer to the traces of very early impressions where the negative associated with speech does not yet have a place. The preverbal inscriptions give form to a past without memory, which can then be transferred into the soma and into action, as an attempt to make psychic materials move on to a new inscription.

A is an educated and refined young woman with a history of traumatic ties maintained with the parental couple, characterised by excesses and affective vexations expressed in a prevailing dynamic of domination and submission experienced since childhood. A's primary objects were not capable of providing an emotional environment suitable for her growth. On the contrary, they required her to constantly conform to their expectations of omnipotent control of her psyche, despite the numerous intellectual resources with which the family was equipped. In a difficult phase of the analysis, the "transferential reawakenings" had turbulently invaded the analytic space and, in the potentiality of transferential repetition, I had become the coercive object of her history, an omnipotent "couple object" laden with potential violence – an invasive foreign body confused with her own self and for this reason difficult to control. At some moments, being in a relationship could be confused with being invaded, drowned. In those instants I felt bound to listen to her emotional turbulences fraught with rage, which provoked a certain malaise in me: one personality might devour the other (Searles 1951). I was experiencing the difficulty of being nailed down in the re-presenting of her transference dynamics, in the psychic place where A needed to position me. In that same phase, at certain painful moments, she was possessed by a compelling necessity for "a motor action" that expressed itself in the urgent need to go to the lavatory, have a "long pee" and so, little by little, calm herself down. She would go back to the couch and could then lie down, recovering a little bit of tranquillity. She had felt very embarrassed the first time and ashamed at revealing the impossibility of containing her "pee full of emotions."

I am aware that such behaviours can be understood in many ways and have many meanings – for example, as an expression of the need to evacuate uncontainable emotional states, or as an externalisation of rage and aggressiveness as a way of attacking the link. However, in our analytic dialogue a new comprehension and working-through of these emergences took shape. We realised together that they distilled multiple levels of inscription in the psyche: my analytic nourishment stirred up intense, almost invasive, affects in her which could immediately re-invest the trace of the invasive, colonising internal object from which a part of herself was not distinct. In those moments, "doing a pee," A felt the urgent need to expel from herself, metaphorically to "spit out," those "nutrients" arising from the encounter with my mind and thus momentarily empty herself (she had suffered from prolonged enuresis in childhood and early adolescence): but this time in the presence of an analyst capable of tolerating her embryonic *No*. It was as if her somatic functions of expulsion potentially contained *a first form of judgement not yet psychically represented*. Such psychic expression needed time to construct an initial subjective appropriation of the nutrients being encountered, meanwhile submitting to an embryonic faculty of judgement expressed in action and the body, which enabled her to decide what to assimilate and what to expel of that "analytic food" she was learning to be nourished by. The opportunity for denial – to refuse the analytic food – was constructing the possibility that A would not have to submit to the coercive repetition of a traumatic link from her history, and that she could try to reappropriate her own mind and her own body by momentarily expressing a *No* that would once have been impossible.

If we widen the forms of analytic listening to make ourselves receptive to the numerous types of communication, we discover that the unconscious speaks many dialects which we can perhaps try to reintegrate into a broader conception of "psychic representation." In it, the "motor gesture" – one of the possible forms of action – may take on a new significance. From this theoretical perspective we entrust the model of the act with the task of gathering up that part of the force of the instinctual-affective motions which it has not been possible to transform into thought; or rather, it has modulated into that heterogeneity of psychic components which proclaim the complexity of relations between affect, the bodily sphere, and the psychic sphere. Unconscious cooperation in the intersubjective space (which includes the intercorporeal levels) is responsible for the first possibility of subjective appropriation and internalisation of these materials.

If we think of memory as a system of multiple signs, the traces of which can be affectively re-invested in various forms depending on the quality of the transferential and countertransferential investments, we must observe that in some cases such traces do not belong to the category of language. From this perspective I would like to suggest that these phenomena should be understood in terms of a "specific form of action" that, to me, seems able to draw on the functions of "the negative" and on forms of listening in which "the negative" can be grasped. In this case it is a question of a negative capable of placing itself beyond the given, as a prefiguring of the subject's ability to become other, of an action that is expressed through a praxis able to transform and create other possible psychic realities. This is the first form of action in which the psyche can decide what to make exist and what to wipe out. (From this viewpoint we should reinterrogate the functions of denial and rejection, in the face of a reality that generates anxiety.)

In *Negation* Freud says, "Judging is the intellectual action which decides the choice of motor action, which puts an end to the postponement due to thought and which leads over from thinking to acting" (Freud 1925a, p. 238). For Freud, to grant or refuse real existence to a representation or a perception (from this perspective, judgement is indeed to be understood as a primal structure in which the qualities of what is good and what is bad take shape, leading to the action of choosing or refusing) would delineate the primary experience understood as instinctual acts of approaching or withdrawing, depending on the phenomena of incorporation-introjection or their repression and rejection. Such an experience would represent the prototype of the earliest instinctual impulses – "'I should like to eat this,' or 'I should like to spit it out'" (Freud 1925a, p. 237).

Expelling and introjecting, denying and affirming can be regarded as operations constituting a primary inner space. In this sense, there is a negative as active work of subjectivity: a first configuration of "psychic action" by means of a *No*, a rejection. This is not expressed on the verbal level but via the body which then becomes the first boundary marker. It is therefore autopoiesis (Varela 1991) that delimits the boundaries of an internal environment where nothing penetrates without being transformed into a compatible form. As if we could suppose an "implicit logic" in a nascent subject (we should remember that the concept of *Verneinung* [denial] is closely contemporary with the first studies of the Ego) in which the psyche can be endowed with forms of response by which to take possession of itself, incorporate, spit out, refuse, reject. All this is to be connected with the effects of pleasure and displeasure provoked from the outset, from the first sensory, perceptual, intero- and exteroceptive experiences.[4] May we speculate that these original features of the Ego or the Self will be preserved as mnemic traces, sensorimotor correlates, which can later be reshaped in new experiences, including those expressed through the use of speech? And will the numerous inscriptions of experiences lived through on the sensory, motor, preverbal, pre-symbolic levels be subsequently translated into verbal expressions and give form to distinctive transferences? Will there be other forms of communication endowed with sense and meaning, capable of expressing affects and emotional states? And again, how are we to capture the essence of an analytic experience that moves off into psychic territories whose functioning reveals a possible impasse with regard to symbolisation? How do we listen to and acknowledge the infinite variations that ultimately concern the fate of the affect in its relations with the bodily and psychic spheres, so that we can distinguish what will be translatable into words from that which will never be?

Let's try focusing on an economic viewpoint, a quantum of affects that we conceive as being intrinsically aimed at communication from the origin of psychic life: affects not in search of discharge (lowering of tension) but in search of another mind able to carry out psychic work of linking and transformation *à deux*. In this view, drive/affect and object are indissociable in their becoming: forms of unconscious cooperation, of polymorphous associativity and co-associativity that draw on those materials ... starting with the traces that they have left behind (Freud 1937).

From my point of view, the economic factor has absolute priority in the investigation of forms of transferential investment and countertransferential listening. We must remember that it is with Ferenczi (1928) that the psychoanalytic set-up has to confront some clinical problems linked to certain types of impasse: the set-up that is offered may produce traumatic repetitions. This focus has facilitated new attention to the matrix of the analyst-patient relationship, to the forms of "psychic work" that need the other, a psychic work *à deux*, when the reverberation of the traumatic register faces us with "an amalgam of heteromorphic psychic materials in which behaviours, acts, bodily sensations, and images are mixed with the verbal forms of the data deriving from perception and sensorimotoricity" (Roussillon 2018, p. 66).

The strength of the affects when listening to certain psychic processes, in their potency which is not yet linked to representations, has a sense of its own. Semiotic acts seeking to be shaped in the transference, force and sense change places and adapt to each other. Since form is inherent in any perception and since perception never perceives itself, sense is already inherent in our perception (Merleau-Ponty 1964). The quantum, an expression of the strength of the affective investment, expresses the feeling which anticipates and maintains thinking, in the same way that poetic language is capable of translating experience and the emotions that accompany it into words endowed with meaning.

So we should ask ourselves: is this perhaps the most profound aspect of that "passionate speech" which is set up between two unconscious voices in the consulting room (Shakespeare, *Hamlet*, II. ii. 427ff: see Fusini 2010) and which, through the "unconscious cooperation" between patient and analyst, can lead to "generative enactments" (Atlas and Aron 2017). A further question arises spontaneously from this: do we need a metapsychology of action?

> I'm always listening to analysts talk about acting-out, and I say to them: "What are you doing about action? Do your patients have actions available to them?" Do you call everything they do acting-out? Psychoanalysts are generally embarrassed because in fact psychoanalysis has no theory of action.
>
> (Green 2005, p. 19)

So, going back once more to consider the affects as an economic whole means adopting a wider perspective on linking and the relationship with the object, but also reassessing the centrality of the body. "The ego is first and foremost a bodily ego" (Freud 1923, p. 26) which, using the basic elements of synchronisation, kinetics, distance, closeness, information about the bodily surface and the movements of the viscera, will subsequently influence language too in its symbolic dimension as a substrate (sensory memory) of affective life: perhaps the earliest poetic register of human life. This is a "vital affective dynamic" able to evoke strength, speed, movement and sense, which may or may not link with elements representing contents: vital forms of feeling that emerge in the first exchanges between mother and baby and constitute the backcloth of the earliest affective fabric. They are founded on the early dual bodily experience, on an intercorporeality that precedes the use of speech and is at the base of subsequent symbolic and metaphorical thought (Stern 2010).

What directions has "our research in the consulting room" taken in recent years? We have attempted to retrace and shed light on an area of psychic functioning and thought that draws its origin from the perceptual-emotional, pre-symbolic, pre-linguistic, and pre-representational levels, and at the same time have taken into account forms of expression of the psychic that involve non-symbolic, non-linguistic, and non-representational registers. We have also understood that the unconscious can express itself in many different forms. As Bollas reminds us, the theory of repression was for a long time the only evidence of unconscious productions, and this did not allow us to observe other forms of unconscious expression, such as unconscious perception, unconscious organisation, and unconscious communication (Bollas 2008).

So, how do we include what we perceive beyond speech among the elements which have significance for our understanding of psychic functioning? In other words, doesn't implicit memory perhaps reveal an emotional schema that follows a logic of its own? Implicit knowing is nowadays considered a sophisticated form of psychic experience of the other that includes affects, expectations and motivations. According to many researchers, this mode of knowledge remains active throughout life and is not replaced by an explicit verbal knowledge. It is a type of "knowing" founded on the experiences that take shape in very distant periods of psychic development and become that affective nucleus of the self from which subsequent symbolic-linguistic transformations will take their starting point (cf. Bollas 1987).

Listening to forms of unconscious intersubjective construction

If, during analytic listening in the session, in that infinite psychic work of provisional construction that happens in our mind, we can extend clinical practice towards comprehending modes of unconscious functioning characterised by limited symbolising functions, we can gain access to new psychoanalytic experiences and increase our capacity for understanding the "subtle interplay" (Winnicott 1986) in which we are engaged. In other words, we find ourselves facing a vast territory created by the "composite structure of the psychic" (Freud 1938a), both conscious and unconscious, determined by the plurality of the traces and temporalities registered in it; between past and future, between what has happened and never been given meaning by the psyche and what has never happened and has only been able to take shape as a negative trace. It is in this crucible that we can re-present heterogeneous forms of expression of the psychic that are capable of conveying communications at a high level of affective intensity, able to make the analyst's psyche resonate in the here and now of the analytic relationship, in specific "work as a double."

In this connection Bion states that

> the intensity of the patient's feelings appears in the analysis as muscular movements, changes in mien, changes in posture, attitude. The feelings are contained in words; the words are not the names of the feelings, but are felt to be the feelings themselves.
>
> (Bion 1992, p. 169)

Let's consider communication between unconsciouses, the functioning of which is temporary, pre-reflective, non-verbal, and non-repressed in character, capable of revealing emotional nuclei in the patient that are excluded from symbolisation. The analyst, Freud reminds us, "must turn his own unconscious like a receptive organ towards the transmitting unconscious of the patient" (Freud 1912, p. 115). This second claim is laden with potential for adding depth to the numerous articulations of the concept of countertransference and the theoretical constructs aimed at taking the role of the analyst's psyche into account when faced with functionings at the boundary.

From a theoretical viewpoint we need to keep in mind, and hold onto as a conceptual background, the move from the first model to the second, from the unconscious to the Id, and from the Id to affect (affective economy). The instinctual impulse, no longer the drive, can be attributed to an economy not only in terms of tensions and discharges but of affects endowed with a semiotic force in search of multiform possibilities for linking in the encounter with the other. Green (1983) reminds us that while in the drive model the work of representation predominates in the attainment of consciousness, in the structural model "it is the strength of the instinctual impulse" that finds space in the form of affect, an affect rooted in the soma, which may find numerous paths for expression, both in symbolic and non-symbolic codes of communication.

The extension of clinical practice has in fact put the theoretical assumptions of our method to the test, giving rise to the requirement that, on the conceptual plane, we take account of what happens between two or more embodied psyches, understanding the psychic in the fullest sense to include forms of expression carried out as action. We have granted such elements a new recognition as highly communicative potential languages and at the same time acknowledged a complexity of elements in verbal productions that have stimulated us to question the ways we listen to the various psychic productions that engage the analytic space. Over time, indeed, as our psychic subject was expanding its own matrices, it was becoming clearer that we need to extend psychoanalytic thinking on the theoretical plane from the sphere of *formulated* thoughts attributable to the dimension of secondary repression, towards the sphere of *unformulated* thoughts. And in order to achieve this extension we needed new theoretical instruments. In relation to this, I would like to recall an observation made as early as 1895 by Freud:

> are we to suppose that we are really dealing with thoughts which never came about, which merely had a *possibility* of existing, so that the treatment would lie in the accomplishment of a psychical act which did not take place at the time?
>
> (Freud 1895, p. 300, italics in original)

Semiotic gestures: "The murmur of things"

Emotional experiences can offer themselves to our comprehension in a motoric guise. Merleau-Ponty reminds us that the body's movements express personal states of mind (Merleau-Ponty 1953).

They are addressed to the other in a form of vital communication, a dynamic interaction made of bodily movements, facial expressions and gestures, revealing the self. There is a motoric accompaniment to the perception of an affective state, gestures revealing registered sensations which testify to the history of singular reverberations from the encounter with the other, able to convey a message that, if it is "named," will reopen these still unformulated psychic movements towards translation into verbal thought. There is, in other words, a "murmur of things" (Merleau-Ponty 1964) that constantly underlies our embodied and affectivised perception, like a warp and weft of potential meanings able, if listened to, to pass along a continuum that goes from the pre-symbolic to the imaginative and all the way to the symbolic (Bucci 1997). It is perhaps the first level of metaphorisation before the acquisition of language, capable of recognising likenesses and differences, and transmitting their meaning (Modell 2009). Using a brief clinical fragment, I will try to describe a particular form of self-expression (Winnicott 1941) by two very different patients at emotionally significant moments in their analytic work; an expressive communication entrusted to a gesture which, once understood at a verbal level, enabled the deeper exploration of certain transferential themes during that period.

In their emotional histories, R and S, a man and a woman, had in common an early encounter with an intrusive, overflowing object which meant that their "idiom" was prematurely and significantly established in rather similar forms. On numerous occasions in a session, during phases of quite substantial transferential investment, as soon as I began to suggest some thoughts, always in carefully chosen words which also revealed my psychic presence as attempting to give form to some kind of understanding, both patients greatly astonished me by making the same, immediate response using a very similar "gesture." They both slightly arched their back, put their arms up and gradually brought them down onto their head, covering it with their hands which they clasped on their neck as if to create a barrier to protect themselves from what might be coming from outside, which was implicitly being likened to a danger, a possible blow. I was deeply struck by how that "gesture," a particular statement expressed directly by a motor action, was trying to transmit a trace registered in a sensorimotor modality, making it present again in the transference. Perhaps it was a first *No* expressed via the body without verbal mediation, a form of communication directed at me in the transference as an affective signal evoking a potential threat. Naturally, my bringing to the centre of analytic attention something that might have remained at the margins, being not communicable in words, allowed the "motor gesture" to be reconnected to a new context of signification and psychic elaboration by means of my "interpretation": an understanding that had nothing to do with a hidden meaning *but with the creation of an absent sense* that had always been left suffering and imprisoned in a motoric schema, having waited perhaps for a long time to be grasped and given meaning through interpretative speech.

A fundamental question: "Investigating the caesura"

The postulate of an embodied psyche is based on the conception of an unconscious rooted in the somatic processes that continually emerge within an intercorporeal and intersubjective matrix and are differentiated into forms of psychic expression along a continuum running from the body to the psyche and returning from the psyche to the body. This continuum is described thus by Freud:

> We know two kinds of things about what we call our psyche (or mental life): firstly, its bodily organ and scene of action, the brain (or nervous system) and, on the other hand, our acts of consciousness, which are immediate data and cannot be further explained by any sort of description. Everything that lies between is unknown to us, and the data do not include any direct relation between these two terminal points of our knowledge.
>
> (Freud 1938a, p. 144)

Therefore, the objective we have been setting ourselves for more than a century is to keep investigating a way of bridging that *caesura*; a way across the immense still unknown territory one step at a time in the attempt to know what lies between the two extremes. In other words, investigate the heterogeneity of the psychic processes of derivation, transformation, and correlation that go from one field of the psyche-soma to the other, in forms that we find to be ever more complex as we try to render them intelligible.

From a conceptual viewpoint, addressing the expressive potentialities of the unconscious, which may articulate itself in multiple and heterogeneous forms, means applying one's listening to the various modes in which the psyche can express itself, "provisionally" reserving the qualities of the conscious for the reflective functions. (In this connection, note the questions raised by authors such as Panksepp, Solms, and Damasio, who attribute the qualities of consciousness to non-reflective functions as well.) These modes run from action to psychic gesture (Sapisochin 2013) and all the way to speech. Given the complexity of clinical registers that we engage with in the consulting room, trying to give an account of the psychic materials with which we come into contact (all "the dialects that our unconscious can utilise") means trying to widen the theoretical spectrum and attempting to investigate the caesuras that still partly inhabit our tools of intelligibility *between body and psyche, thing and word, pre-symbolic and symbolic, preverbal and verbal, etc.* In this brief theoretical survey I will consider some landmarks from Freud's own journey, more specifically from early and late Freud, against a background of the theory of the living body at the base of the evolutions of post-Freudian metapsychologies which continue in various ways to investigate the birth and formation of the psychic structures within embodied relational matrices.

In this brief conceptual exploration I will start with the concept of *Agieren* which Freud uses for the first time in the case of Dora (for a fuller examination, see Turillazzi Manfredi and Pazzagli 1986). We find ourselves faced with a dramatisation of affect, an affect returning to life and unable to express itself in words, but only through the dynamics of recollection: the subject "reproduces it not as a memory but as an action; he *repeats* it, without, of course, knowing that he is repeating it" (Freud 1914a, p. 150). The first question would be, what characteristic of the unconscious was Freud describing when he attributed to it the property of repetition as action "without knowing that he is repeating it"?

The contemporary conception of the unconscious presupposes the ability to preserve the traces of the numerous forms of inscription, to carry out affective re-investments and new transcriptions (Edelman 1990 would say re-categorisations), and to produce expressions that communicate affective states. Such communicative expressions run from the first sensorimotor experiences and the interoceptive states to verbal exchanges. (I am alluding to the sonic, linguistic and gestural immersion that the infant shares in the interchange with the primary environment where its experiences take shape.) In his late works, such as the *Outline of Psychoanalysis*, but also earlier in *The Ego and the Id*, Freud proposes the hypothesis that "representations of something" may become conscious not only through speech, but also through an image or a representation of movement. From this perspective, language is not the only means by which the unconscious can become conscious: this may be achieved via multiple expressive avenues. Nevertheless, a genuinely reflective consciousness will only be able to reveal itself in language or, to put it another way, in the "hearing of hearing" (knowing of knowing). In this connection, Bion wonders,

> Can any method of communication be sufficiently "penetrating" to pass that caesura in the direction from post-natal conscious thought back to the pre-mental in which thoughts and ideas have their counterpart in "times" or "levels" of mind where they are not thoughts or ideas?
>
> (Bion 1977, p. 45)

Or should we suppose a "thought without language"? – keeping in mind, with Bion, a delicate theme of temporality in which he reminds us, "One cannot go back ... It is in the present that we have to *have a method of formulation which can penetrate the barrier*" (Bion 1977, p. 47, my italics). *But couldn't we metaphorically penetrate such a barrier by actualising the traces inscribed in the memory via various communicative codes?*

Following this line of thought, it seems essential to go beyond the caesura – between those forms of unconscious registering which structure psychic development on the pre-symbolic and pre-linguistic level – and investigate the way in which the advent of the symbolic-linguistic capacities re-invest these traces, and the type of psychic work to which they are subjected. As we continue to explore the relationships between the psyche's various forms of expression, what we can assert – as Loewald (1980) reminds us – is that the beginnings of language must not be thought of as a sort of *translation* of sensory experience but as a form of *sensory* experience:

> While the mother utters words, the infant does not perceive words but is bathed in sound, rhythm, etc., as accentuating ingredients of a uniform experience ... Words ... embody [a thing] in a specific sensory-motor medium. The sensory-motor elements of speech remain bodily ingredients of language ... This aspect continues to dwell in language, although unattended to, even in its most abstract use, and in written and read language and "inner speech" as well.
>
> (Loewald 1980, pp. 187 and 203)

So words function as a creative vehicle in "a creative act similar to that in poetry, where language is found for phenomena, contexts, connections, experiences not previously known and speakable" (Loewald 1980, p. 242). We should recall that Stern, by contrast, holds that the infant's preverbal and verbal experiences are separated by a hiatus and, though he conceptualises the sense of a preverbal self, he believes that the development of language sacrifices the sensory and sensual richness of preverbal experience:

> But in fact language is a double-edged sword. It also makes some parts of our experience less shareable with ourselves and with others. It drives a wedge between two simultaneous forms of interpersonal experience: as it is lived and as it is verbally represented. Experience in the domains of emergent, core, and intersubjective relatedness, which continue irrespective of language, can be embraced only very partially in the domain of verbal relatedness.
>
> (Stern 1985, p. 162)

Keeping an additional perspective in the background, we have learned in dialogue with the neuroscientific disciplines that our perception is shaped by action, even when we are not carrying out a movement, and that action represents an original, primary way of being involved in the world around us. The discovery in the brain's motor areas of neurons that are activated by simply observing another person's intentional, directed actions (an embodied simulation at the foundation of the imaginative processes) has provided neurophysiological bases for psychoanalytic observations about the subject's capacity for assimilating another person's internal state. This assimilation does not only pass along the paths of reflectiveness and symbolic representation but also through pre-reflective mimetic openings which are much more direct and automatic, whose mediation is corporeal; "imitating in order to be" (Gaddini 1969). Discoveries like these have resonated with the research of contemporary psychoanalysis into the concepts of empathy, imitation, and identification, unconscious communication and projective identification. The mirroring mechanisms are considered to be the basis for constructing a primitive bodily self-awareness which precedes and underlies any reflective self-awareness (Gallese and Sinigaglia 2010). For Freud, from the *Project* onwards, both perception between self and outside world and between self and internal bodily perceptions (in other words, the exteroceptive and interoceptive modes) are founded on unconscious processes that need no translation into words (although translation into words will change their physiognomies and their tasks): psychoanalysis "explains the supposedly somatic concomitant phenomena as being what is truly psychical, and thus in the first instance disregards the quality of consciousness" (Freud 1938a, p. 158). In a note written on a sheet of paper in 1938 from his exile in London, he left us a fascinating and enigmatic assertion: "Psyche is extended; knows nothing about it" (included among the notes of "Findings, ideas, problems" in the final volume of the collected works).

As we follow this route, we are aware that Freud's thinking from the outset presents us with twin tracks: on the one hand, the centrality of language, representation in words, the *talking cure*, in the concept of therapeutic action; and on the other, *the revelation of the non-linguistic nature of the unconscious*: a living unconscious that is the background of all Freud's work and is broadened and extended in several later theoretical developments. I am thinking for example of Winnicott, who never separates his conception of psychoanalytic functioning from what he calls the psyche-soma, from the sensory experience in which the mind takes shape:

> To study the concept of mind one must always be studying an individual, a total individual, and including the development of that individual from the very beginning of psychosomatic existence. If one accepts this discipline then one can study the mind of an individual as it specialises out from the psyche part of the psyche-soma.
>
> The mind does not exist as an entity in the individual's scheme of things provided the individual psyche-soma or body scheme has come satisfactorily through the very early developmental stages; mind is then no more than a special case of the functioning of the psyche-soma …
>
> I suppose the word psyche here means the *imaginative elaboration of somatic parts, feelings, and functions*, that is, of physical aliveness.
>
> (Winnicott 1949, p. 244, italics in original)

From the viewpoint outlined here, the unconscious is not only structured like a language but is hypothesised as a function able to transcribe simultaneous forms of experience: the lived and the verbally represented. The former keeps a trace of itself in time through a number of mnemic codes while the latter captures the present moment, again using several registers, in some cases different from the verbal or parallel to it: a semiotic unconscious capable of utilising all the levels of the psyche-soma to communicate.

So we should go back and ask ourselves: how do we listen out for and acknowledge the infinitely varied fate of affect in its relations with the bodily and psychic spheres so as to distinguish what will be translatable into words from what will never be, but instead will continue to inhabit the psyche in the form of the unsayable?

All sensations play a part in the expression of emotional movements consisting originally of "suitable acts" and "specific actions."

> There can be no doubt that [the psychic] apparatus has only reached its present perfection after a long period of development ... The exigencies of life confront it first in the form of the major somatic needs. The excitations produced by internal needs seek discharge in movement, which may be described as an "internal change" or an "expression of emotion." A hungry baby screams or kicks helplessly. But the situation remains unaltered, for the excitation arising from an internal need is not due to a force producing a *momentary* impact but to one which is in continuous operation. A change can only come about if in some way or other (in the case of the baby, through outside help) an "experience of satisfaction" can be achieved which puts an end to the internal stimulus.
>
> (Freud 1899, p. 565)

If, therefore, in the first link and the vital urgency of an affective communication the first communication is established by means of motility, it will later be the source from which language will arise. Thus the affect will be linked, on the one hand, to the communicative function – i.e. to language – and, on the other hand, to bodily experience through which the specific action of the nearest human being is solicited. The languages of flesh and of speech draw on a common source. The drive/affect is located between body and language. The urge to psychically elaborate an event that has aroused a strong impression may manifest itself through repetition in play, but that which is unpleasant may assume other forms. The character of repetition coexists with great psychic intensities and shows itself to be independent of the organisation of the other psychic processes which is what allows us to live reality.

In conclusion, based on these observations, what it seems important to me to emphasise is that we should take a wider psychic field into consideration, a psyche-soma, the signs and landmarks of which belong to multiple codes of registration and communication. They transition across the various registers of our functioning: intrapsychic, intersubjective, interpsychic, and intercorporeal. Such a widening of perspective naturally has repercussions for the way we conceive therapeutic action. The historic work of the Boston Change Process Study Group, *The "Something More" Than Interpretation*, has revealed that many changes during analysis do not only occur as the consequence of conscious insights, but also as the consequence of experiences of interaction – moments of meeting, non-verbal and behavioural cognitive forms in the field of the procedural unconscious – between analyst and patient. Paraphrasing the title of the BCPSG report, it would in my opinion be helpful to continue reflecting on *something more than speech or more than what is in speech*. While language allows us to share some aspects of our experiences with others, we all know from our own analysis and numerous experiences with our patients how limited speech can be. Indeed, language is also the agency that separates the primary and secondary processes from each other, and makes parts *left out* of our experience become "less shareable with ourselves and with others" (Stern 2010). Experience which happens in the field of the relationship between two subjects according to a multiplicity of codes (Bucci 1997) can only partly be made to re-enter the field of verbal relations. To the extent that only events occurring in the field of verbal relations are considered to have "reality," a significant part of psychic experience, the body included, may become the submerged field of experience (Stern 2010).

Listening to excess: "That nothing, that too much." A different reflection on the dimensions of the traumatic

Let's return to traumatic intensities. If excess is posited as that which cannot be symbolised or held in dialogic mental space (Benjamin 2017), then research on trauma becomes a matter of paying attention to the conditions that foster or prevent the development of psychic life. From this viewpoint, it becomes necessary to adopt a complex perspective, free from reductionism and linear casualisms: indeed, although the historical and the psychic intricately overlap with each other, they do not coincide. So it is a viewpoint that tries hard to delineate affective facts and experiences in order to comprehend *the difficult complexity of the dialogue between psyche and event*. Indeed, we use "traumatic" to define the occurrence that has surprised and overwhelmed the psyche, the threat of intrusion to which it has been exposed, an event that it has not been possible to deal with by means of representation and symbolisation: experiences from which we are protected in various ways, chiefly to preserve our continuity of being (Roussillon 2002); psychic traces which inhabit the internal world as systems of subterranean life that constantly parasitise the subject's psyche. It is a thoroughgoing system of traumatic memories which strive to be represented, to burst into the present, into the analytic scenario, with the aim of involving another mind in order to integrate these experiences in a possible subjective appropriation, as a rudimentary experience of "me." Such traces can be combined in the forms of the various memory systems described by Freud (Bastianini 2002): traces revealing signs, perceptions linked to experiences which endure in forms of affective registration that irrupt into life as unnameable fears, states of despair and loneliness.

Naturally, we are thinking of the shadow of the object that falls on the Ego – an Ego that in the beginning is bodily above all – and the many complex traces it can leave in its indelible imprint, revealing the quality *of the object's presence in constant dialogue with the subject's unconscious creativity*. What happens is important, but even more significant is what the happening will become, what the infantile psyche will make of it, in what way it will be able to reconnect itself with the rest of psychic life. From this perspective, it becomes fundamental to rethink *the forms of subjective appropriation in all their possible permutations*. Experiences and meanings, the impressions received at the origin of psychic life – pleasant or unpleasant, traumatic or generative – cannot in fact be ignored by the psyche. They must be integrated, represented, symbolised.

Let's keep asking ourselves what enables a human being to escape the repetition, and especially traumatic repetition, of their own history.[5] What is repeated are often experiences that could not be integrated; experiences occurring in early periods when the infant psyche was not yet capable of performing integrative functions. In his final hypotheses about repetition, Freud no longer refers to the death instinct but to integration or non-integration; at the end of his life it is this latter topic which assumes a fundamental role. Later it was Winnicott who clarified how, within the transitional space, the mind's integrative functions, if adequately supported, create the fundamental conditions for the integrative process in the psychic space.

For a long time psychoanalysis has been enquiring into the impact that adverse experiences can have on the sense of continuity of existence, the sources of which can be numerous and different for each individual. Thanks to the prominence given to the functions of the primary object and the related concepts of holding, handling, and reverie, the contributions of psychoanalytic authors in the second half of the last century have brought about a shift of interest from traumas "of excess" to traumas "of deficit." While in the origin of psychoanalytic thought the excesses of excitation and the "confusion of tongues" by the adult in relation to the child were the central elements, the years that followed saw a growing interest in traumas caused by deficiency – of holding (Winnicott 1965), for example, or in the function of reverie (Bion 1962) – which has culminated in what has been called, especially since Green, "clinical work on the void" (Green 2002). A further, related field of research into the injuries suffered by the feeling of self, into the role played by illusion in the "found-created," or the loss of an object with distinctive mirroring functions, such as Kohut's "selfobject" (1971), constitutes a parallel way to comprehend failings in the subject's relationship with reality and the resulting loss of sense. Once again, a sense is recorded, albeit in negative, which endures in the psyche and waits for a potential re-investment.

What happens to the psyche when early disinvestment and excess of excitation disturb the psychic work of linking, elaboration, and symbolisation? There is a predominance of psychic functions that aim to detach the subject's psyche from external reality, producing a separate area *not integrated* with the rest of experience

(Williams 2009). When the painful reality is also only partly eclipsed by psychic reality, the individual's self-awareness is damaged: the psychic work of linking affect and representation is blocked; a caesura is created in the feeling of self.

At the end of *Moses and Monotheism*, besides recognising among the reasons for traumatic experiences "also ... early injuries to the ego (narcissistic mortifications)" (Freud 1934–1938, p. 74), Freud stresses that the effects of the trauma may be of two types: positive and negative. The former lead to the compulsion to repeat; but it is in the second, in the negative aspect, that the journey starts to be made in search of phenomena of emptiness, symptoms without content, memories without recollection – that is, to phenomena laid down at the foundation of the traumatic, in that dimension where it is impossible to transform the experiences which could not be the object of a psychic work of translation, representation, and symbolisation. Moreover, in 1938, returning in "Constructions in Analysis" to the conditions that trigger delirium and hallucinations, Freud once again evokes the subjective experiences that precede the appearance and use of the apparatus of language.

The existence of such traces seems likely to have been inflicted in the "negative of trauma": a void paradoxically filled with negative links that disconnect affect from the possibilities of representation, a negative that makes the work of mourning and repression impossible (Botella and Botella 2001; Green 2002). Not being transformable by the psychic work that leads to symbolisation, the traumatic dimension persists in psychic life as the sign of something fundamental which cannot be remembered or forgotten: *an impasse that produces "memories without recollection"* (Bastianini and Moccia 2003). As if in a psychic suspension, the traumatic area cannot be connected to inside or outside. Unable to be transformed in the network of representations, conflicts, investments and counterinvestments, it remains encysted in the psyche as a sign of something fundamental that has not yet been thought by the subject (Bollas 1987; Winnicott 1971).

How do we listen to the outcomes of such vicissitudes, which may be located at the limits of psychic subjectivity? Indeed, a desertification of the unrepresentable psychic fabric comes to be created, accompanied by "primary defence reactions," "restriction of the Ego," "states of splitting-dissociation of the Ego." As Roussillon reminds us, "In the exploration of the reasons that impel the ego-subject to alter itself, distort itself, or break apart, the question of trauma occupies an essential place" (Roussillon 2006, p. 77). In fact, trauma leaves pervasive traces, conceptualised as alienating influences (Aulagnier 1979; Faimberg 2005; Kaës et al. 1993) characterised by a distinctive narcissistic economy producing bonds that put psychoanalytic practice to the test in the tyrannical repetition of traumatic affective states. It is as well to remember that these repetitions contain the paradox of a new attempt made by the subject, through the use of another psyche, to try to integrate and symbolise areas of the mind that are waiting to be led towards new forms of psychic existence.

So we are dealing with "psychic intensities" capable of investing in the ways the analyst listens and making them resonate in equally complex forms. In *Analysis Terminable and Interminable* Freud emphasises that emotional contiguity with the patient's "repressed material" may lead to "dangers" for the analyst (1937, p. 249), almost a risk of illness. That is, the patient's unconscious may mobilise various forms of affective investment, determining ways of listening that involve numerous registers of the analyst's psyche-soma. So the consulting room becomes a laboratory in which to cultivate a readiness to research the most suitable ways of creating the conditions whereby "an analytic experience" can take shape. It becomes fundamental to ask oneself how to listen to and recognise the infinite possible outcomes that can befall the affect in its relations with the bodily and psychic spheres, so that we can try to distinguish what will be translatable into words from what will never be.

From a metapsychological viewpoint, this means continuing to look "in the living discourse" (Green 1973), the complex relationship between the paths of verbal symbolisation and those of affective symbolisation, for evidence of the quality of the encounter between the subject's unconscious creativity and the "transformative objects" of experience (Bollas 2008). To try and delineate the trajectories of a psyche that may be expressed in a range of communicative registers, we must once again aim to widen the boundaries of psychoanalytic treatment, which is being pushed ever further towards early regions of psychic development where the object's response can leave an indelible imprint: holes in the fabric of representations, lacunae in the affective investments. Psychic conditions where there is no room for a distinction between tolerable absence (registered against a background of presence and hence symbolisable) and the impossibility of working through the painful psychic experience in which emptiness becomes the only (and paradoxical) sign of a fullness to cling to, in which "all I have got is what I have not got," as a patient put it to Winnicott (1971). We are faced with an unprecedented dialectical articulation of the "aspects of the negative" which take shape between the psychic dimensions of absence, loss, and emptiness (Green 2002). Traumatic traces which are translated into anxieties and disturbances of the processes of symbolisation and subjectivation, emotional states inexpressible on the symbolic and metaphorical level, affective turbulences that can only "be made present" in the body, in action, or in the resonances of enactment.

The body knows: Brief clinical reflections

How do we gain access to what is communicated but not represented in words?

F is a psychotherapist trying to deal with a painful moment in her life. In a session from her training analysis, she tells me about one of her patients who has constant thoughts of suicide, and the terrible headache that she herself had suffered during the most recent psychotherapy session as she was listening powerlessly to the monotonous, hopeless speech of her patient. F points out that, in contrast with so many previous sessions that had lacked emotional resonance, on this occasion the patient had begun to talk about the traumatic loss of her husband (from a devastating stroke; she had heard him gasping for breath). To her surprise, F had observed that as she was listening to her patient's painful story, her headache started to fade until it disappeared altogether. While she is struggling to recount this episode, she incredulously lets me know that the headache is assailing her once again, and yet, in an equally astonishing and mysterious way, the headache had vanished instantly when the associating patient prompted the recovery of a memory from when F was 10 years old and had learned about the traumatic death of her grandfather: was it perhaps a heart attack? Or something else that had been kept from her? She recalled with irritation and pain the way the news had been communicated to her: brutally, baldly, with no protection for her young mind. The experience of feeling emotionally neglected by her own family had been a constant in F's life throughout her childhood years. She recalls how on that occasion she felt a chill run through her. *A frost fell over her emotions and she no longer felt that she was fully in herself:* an experience of depersonalisation and dissociation that would accompany many later moments in F's life. Listening to her words, I am drawn in and curious, but at the same time feel a sense of unease, an almost physical malaise. What is happening in the consulting room? What psychic field has been formed between F and her patient, and now between us? *What symmetries and resonances with past experiences can have given rise on the intercorporeal level to an unconscious communication in which the psychotherapist's body has become the site for the recording of affects that have not yet been verbally symbolised?* (A pervasive experience on the intrapsychic plane inserted into the intersubjective and/or intercorporeal space with the aim of regulating its painful intensity.) Reflecting *après-coup* on the phenomena brought by the patient and repeated in action in the transference, I formulated the hypothesis that, in an enactment, F had undergone with her patient the unconsciously shared *repetition in action* of an "affective record" during childhood in her own environment, based on the need to preserve her mind through an early dissociation of affective states. In those precise moments, the headache signalled the temporary loss of the functions for working on her emotions, whereas in her own session it could have had meaning as an enacted transference communication about the same dissociative dynamics that she was afraid of repeating in the relationship with her analyst. On this occasion too, the expansion of the narrative envelope, making it able to grasp and give meaning to the forms of communication between analyst and patient, had enabled unconscious work as a couple which made a working-through possible instead of a repetition. The mutually constructed intercorporeal psychic field indicated substantial symmetries in the field of lived experiences and of the unconscious solutions adopted for dealing with them. The presence of another mind (F's as therapist, and mine in F's training session) was able to perform an immediate function of containing and transforming the dissociated affect, so as to render it communicable and thus reduce its power to cause anxiety, giving rise to a new interpsychic field.

G is a seasoned professional, in analysis for problems at work and in his personal relationships caused by a limited ability to contain internal conflicts which stop him from being able to assert himself in front of others; concomitant states of anxiety that generate panic attacks frequently punctuate his daily life. He would never let himself go enough to make an explicit expression of anger, and yet one of his problems is that he is subjected to bullying by others. Over time, it becomes clear how his tendency to passivity is a defence against anxiety, which he feels every time interpersonal situations of potential conflict arise. G arrives for his session and starts talking light-heartedly about something that has not turned out well at work. Then he abruptly changes the subject and tells me that some hours before, while he was on the spinning machine at the gym, the monitor was showing a film of highly intense fighting (a battle between Asians going all out against each other). To his great astonishment he discovers that as he watches the film, his pedalling rate goes up by twenty units. This worries him and he immediately gets off the machine. During the session he makes a joke about his mirror neurones (which are part of the jargon we share) having perhaps imprisoned him in an experience where his anger had found a way of expressing itself for the first time by using "the Asians." In the session we reconstruct the fact that the anger, of which he had been unaware at that moment, had found a first chance to reveal itself in direct, bodily form as he watched the fight between the Asians. It was only at a later moment, with the help of the analytic work, that it was possible for him to recognise and subjectively appropriate his own aggressive feelings about certain colleagues who had manipulated and betrayed him, and now he could attribute all this to an oedipal dynamic that had never "waned"!

Countertransference, enactment, subjectivity and intersubjectivity, or rather "intersubjective field," are constructs that have acquired their own status, becoming part of several theoretical paradigms. The neurosciences' discovery of implicit memory's neural circuits (Kandel 1999; LeDoux 1996) has conferred a biological basis on the psychoanalytic inferences about the memory of the affects, which is older than the cognitive and symbolic memory, and persists as a lifelong trace influencing the cognitive operations and the elaborating of information. Indeed, we know today that in the first three years of life infantile experiences are registered in a pre-symbolic code in the circuits of the implicit memory, with a wide role in constituting a different form of unconscious from the dynamic repressed unconscious. Such experiences can be transcribed as emotional schemata of unconscious meanings dissociated from the child's self-perception, and yet they have the power to influence psychic experience, the effects of which are not understood. A schema of unconscious meanings is constructed, providing a code for the constant evaluation of experiences and sensations so that they can be internalised. But this code does not belong to the integrated experience of the self: the psychic work that it compels is a constant need to organise experience in a form that helps to maintain this exclusion (Klein 1976; Ogden 2016). Dissociation (for brevity I won't rehearse what has been said in other contexts about the use of the term in relation to the concept of splitting, as for example by Ferenczi, 1928) is a strategy for emotional survival that is activated very early in life, allowing traumatic affects to be managed, *flight when there is nowhere to flee to* (Putnam 1997).[6] When the reflective functions fail to contain intense emotions, these are expelled from awareness (cf. Freud's concept of *Verwerfung* and its subsequent integrations and evolutions) and the field is taken by the body, which is left to bear solitary witness to the psychic pain. The syntonic and empathic responses of the child's caregivers enable the development of the affects, which are experienced in the beginning as bodily sensations and later in subjective states that can be communicated by speech (Krystal 1988). We have, moreover, become increasingly aware that traumatic experiences profoundly influence the levels of reflective functioning and determine the failure of elaboration on the symbolic plane:

> Part of the medium through which early trauma makes its imprint on the psychic-soma is through the establishment of a dissociated memory system in which experiences of the disruption of self experience are stored in a form that cannot be processed as one's own past thoughts, feelings, perceptions, bodily sensations, and so on. Rather, these unthinkable thoughts and feelings that cannot be felt intrude into consciousness as unaccountable and often unnameable states of fear, despair, loneliness, dread and the like and intrude into the body as psychosomatic disorders.
>
> (Ogden 2000, p. x)

We have learned that the body *knows* and can "keep the score" (Van der Kolk 2014) in place of the psyche: "Affective states are incorporated into the life of the psyche as precipitates of primal traumatic experiences, and are evoked in similar situations like memory symbols" (Freud 1925b, p. 622).

"Dissociated" places in the mind: Flight when there is nowhere to flee to

> This patient said: "At the beginning the individual is like a bubble. If the pressure from outside actively adapts to the pressure within, then the bubble is the significant thing, that is to say the infant's self. If, however, the environmental pressure is greater or less than the pressure within the bubble, then it is not the bubble that is important but the environment. The bubble adapts to the outside pressure."
>
> (Winnicott 1949, pp. 182–183)

P is a brilliant and intelligent young artist. He is only able to stay in the analytic space as long as he can enchant/hypnotise the analyst with his fantastical oratory or, alternatively, by escaping from himself and the other person by withdrawing into his inner world. Stretched out on the couch, after some exchanges that were very engaging on the emotional level, he puts his hands on his head. Like a prisoner in front of the enemy. As if he had to protect himself from a possible blow. He plunges into a profound silence: he is somewhere else, he has fled. As if in the implicit state of the analytic relationship an excess of intimacy had occurred, a psychic conjunction held for too long, which he must interrupt so that he can flee into the interior places that shelter and protect him: his *psychic retreat* (Steiner 1993).

A retreat where he is detached from himself in order to create a distance from the other who has invaded him. He flees from himself as a bulwark against the overflowing "of the other" into him.

One day, during a rather laborious session, perhaps enacting my impatience after one of his "flights," I ask him almost impulsively, but also following a vague intuition, "Where are you? Are you here? Or have you gone somewhere else?" At that difficult juncture I was privately wondering about his emotional atlas, his secret psychic geography from which I felt totally excluded. Then, in my reverie there appeared the memory of Pirandello's story *Geography is the Remedy* which I had read some time before. It was as if at that precise moment I had been able to bring together all the internal and external data "into a single intelligible unity aimed at binding all the heterogeneous elements that are present into an atemporal simultaneity" (Botella and Botella 2001, p. 48). The story's protagonist, who has to watch over his old, dying mother, finds himself almost in a trance state, not knowing how much time has passed, not feeling "tiredness, cold, or despair," with a geography book of his daughter's lying open at a page showing a map of Jamaica. For some unspecified time he had been on that island, in the Blue Mountains, among pleasant hills and broad sunlit valleys. The protagonist goes on to give a highly vivid description of fantastic places, as if ecstatically carried away, an abduction by places that fills him with sensations. He clings to these "new havens" so that he can escape a real one that is too painful to bear.

I am using Pirandello's story[7] to illustrate a spatial metaphor I had found helpful in "comprehending" the vicissitudes of a principal mode of psychic work in trauma: the possibility for the subject to relocate himself protectively in another psychic place, dissociating from the painful experience of himself, as P did with his ways of being with me in the consulting room which confronted me with the paradox of a *relationship of non-relationship* (Green 2002).

P goes away, detaches himself from me, in an attempt to anaesthetise and isolate the pain and reach an elsewhere, another psychic place where the geography is mysterious; the only remedy for the distressing fear that he will rediscover traces of the traumatic object from his past in the transference. The imagination has the task of saturating a potentially fragmenting psychic experience: he "feels with his imagination and not with his heart" (Pessoa 2016).

He is struck by the question "where are you, are you still here?" It is as if he has woken from a dream, perhaps he is also relieved, and asks how I came to realise this: nobody else seems to have found out how he absents himself and goes off to his secret places. He clearly sees for the first time, with astonishment, that in his conversation he often finds himself inhabiting a retreat, especially with women who engage him emotionally. He dissimulates his absence by adopting a false self as a perfect gentleman. This allows him to seduce them and win them over before inwardly abandoning them while remaining physically present.

During his childhood, as we reconstruct it in the session, P discovered that he could relocate himself in an elsewhere, distance himself from a reality that hurt him; over time he learned to reproduce this apparently lifesaving affective schema in every significant relationship. He learned when he was very young to partially dissolve every link with reality and then recreate it in his elsewhere-world where he could protect himself against the encounter with the intrusive, entangling "objects" that sometimes brutally imposed themselves, robbing him of his individuality. It is in the environment he grew up in, and in its deficits, among figures incapable of acknowledging his feelings, that we find the roots of this inability to feel that he is the author of his own life, master of his own affective investments.

The primitive personal memory, used in a magical way, was helping to sustain the functioning of the Self in its omnipotent-omniscient expansion: an imaginary spatiotemporal dimension produced by his fantasying which was seemingly saving him from a pervasive feeling of annihilation. Outwardly, he was giving a part of his mind as a sop to the object using the affability of the false self, attempting to safeguard something of his deepest "idiom," trying to keep it whole, secret, and partially alive in his retreat. The defensive dissociation had this purpose: that is, it was an activity directed towards psychological survival, saving at least that part of his Self, however partial and precarious, that he was in a position to construct and preserve despite the serious insufficiencies of his originating matrix.

Encounters with patients like P show that the forms of subjective appropriation need another mind if they are to be experienced. This means "living witnesses" who can comprehend the need for flight from oneself as an indispensable defence mechanism for survival. From this perspective, the analyst must never stop picturing them beyond the defensive-adaptive structure: in other words, picture them from the perspective of a future in which their idiom will at last be revealed, integrated, recognised and accepted. It is the analyst who can assume the functions that the environment is not able to perform and, by following the scars and the psychic repairs that the subject has been able to carry out, can rediscover the highly traumatic quality of a subject–object relationship founded on non-recognition and exclusion (Cahn 2002).

Listening to "the blue note": Reflections on the COVID-19 period

I will offer some thoughts about a specific form of traumatism that we lived through in this dramatic period. I have felt it incumbent on me not to avoid making such reflections as I can about the distressing times that have had such an impact on our lives, including our professional life. So I would like to suggest some observations about a clinical exchange that took place just after the first lockdown began – a dramatic moment for us all, which tested and continues to test our psychic and therapeutic fitness.

During the pandemic we had to learn to live with the anxieties it caused, and with the time needed to overcome it. We understand more and more clearly and painfully that there will be no mythical "fresh start" in which everything will "magically" go back to the way it was before. Indeed, sometimes our psyche oscillates between the desire to turn our back on the dramatic event and a simultaneous eagerness to imagine a future whose form we do not yet know, and we understand ever more clearly that not everything will be like the past. It is dizzying to try and keep such contradictory and conflicting impulses together as they occupy our minds. We have had to learn, step by step, from our individual experience and that of the human community to which we belong, the ways and forms that may be necessary at the various levels of our coexistence, human, social and professional. How do we rediscover forms of neighbourliness, closeness to fellow members of our species, qualities that are fundamental, indispensable elements in the construction of our humanity, and at the same time learn to contain the anxiety about possible contagion? And what about our "living laboratory," our "kaleidoscopic room" where two flesh-and-blood people talk, two embodied psyches take shape and are mutually transformed? What is left of that?

What elements are in play and must be managed in the abrupt transformation of our internal setting and our usual frame of reference, which required us to "switch to remote" when dealing with unconscious forms of communication that were waiting for our psychic work "as a double" in order to take shape? We have discovered how tiring it is to spend hours every day on the telephone with patients, trying together to recreate an environment of adequate safety and privacy. In my experience, the main psychic work was to make myself available for a new kind of listening, alert to the nuances of the voice so as to catch the rhythm, the prosody of the psychic productions, those fragments of unconscious life communicated by words; words charged with psychic intensities that wander around the room, inside me, in my imagination and my memory. Where are they to go? We cannot yet say where with any certainty, but what I can assert is that such exchanges have in any case been able to set my imagination in motion.

In the attempt to extend the metapsychological boundaries of psychoanalytic listening, I will make use of a remarkable suggestion offered by the brilliant young professional B, at the start of the dramatic pandemic and the subsequent lockdown. This painfully alienating experience, which suddenly exposed us, both in our private lives and our professional activity, to the loss of every familiar point of reference, was accompanied by the need to find solutions that would, as far as possible, safeguard some form of continuity in the relationship with our patients. In this emotional atmosphere, after making the difficult decision to conduct sessions with B remotely, by voice alone and without pictures, near the end of the first session he suggested that "Maybe *we too* have to listen to our blue note!" Surprised and disoriented by this statement, and also curious about it, I wondered what he was alluding to in his sibylline sentence which evoked a psychic space identified by a "we": "The blue note," a musical sign to which a colour is attributed? Inside a sound a micro-melody can be discovered that proclaims a tension which is experienced in the whole body (Merleau-Ponty 1945), and the way I listened was immediately caught by the sensory qualities of the two words: blue, note. I did not yet know the meaning of the expression or its historical origins. At that moment, as my mind resonated with B, I found myself thinking about an invitation received around the same time. This was an invitation to listen to a piece by Miles Davis called *Blue in Green*. It came from a friend whose father was a noted artist (his research as a painter developed against the background of many different elements from the culture of his time, including jazz). The invitation offered a connection between the music and some visual artworks. I had listened to the music that morning, following my friend's instructions, and at that moment in the communication between B and me the multiple connotations of "blue" came to the front of my mind in a sort of mnemic synaesthesia of forms, images, sounds and colours. In my thoughts I associated the blues to the songs of African American slaves, and to the connotations of the term *blue* in English: sadness, nostalgia, loss. I was meditating on the strength and evocative intensity of those musical movements, their vital rhythm; a heartrending song in which several voices can conjoin and separate in rapid sequences, giving life to a characteristic musical polyphony. Perhaps this is what was happening to my imagination as I listened to B's words, which had triggered an abrupt chain of associations. *Après-coup*, I understood how those associations had been fostered by an affective background we both shared – the pain, sadness and nostalgia for a familiar world from which we had been expelled with traumatic violence – and we did not know if and how we would be able to find it again in the future: our "meeting paradigm." B's associative words represented the first affective movement in which a young man's hopes and fears were being distilled. At that moment he was directing a communication towards another psyche's listening, *"towards the symbolising listening of the analyst,"* in the expectation that those words could be "opened" to their original trace, or rather their plurality of traces (Fédida 2012), so that they could be regenerated in new openings up of sense.

I understand later what B means by a "blue note." We are in France during the summer of 1846, in George Sand's pleasant country house where Chopin and other famous intellectuals of the period (Delacroix, Dumas *fils*, Turgenev) were guests. Summer evenings enriched by the Polish musician's improvised recitals which (so we are told in Delacroix's notes) concluded with an almost inaudible note that only George Sand was able to recognise: the blue note, as it was called by Sand herself or by Delacroix as they listened to Chopin play. Such a note would represent the potential of a sound, evoked by a previous musical movement, to recall a suspended note that captures the listener's attention in a remarkable way. It is a note which, as it is listened to, reveals an emotion of recognition: it arrives surprisingly since it remains suspended, we could say, between "the two psyches in reciprocal listening." At the same time, since it does not exist in itself, such a note can be fleeting and suddenly dissolved.

What was B trying to communicate by his enigmatic metaphor with its specific timing? After all, we were nearly at the end of the session. Was he perhaps alluding to the need for us, in our remote relationship, to look for a listening aimed at identifying psychic movements within our expectation of other "sounds" that can evoke a sense capable of revealing itself beyond the words themselves? All of this in a temporality that was occupying space in the bustle of my mind, well after the end of the session. (In that critical moment, I found myself recalling the words of

M, a young professional woman with whom I was then discovering the complexity of remote listening, without images: "I can hear you smiling.")

My associative psychic work had linked B's metaphor to a theme of loss, nostalgia, and pain, in which the "blues singing" of African American slaves, taken by violence far from their birthplaces, became a powerful evoker of "psychic intensities" experienced in the here and now of our remote session.

During these months, immersed in the distressing and pervasive sensation of being on the threshold of a catastrophe for humanity, we were coping with uncertainty, the feeling of crisis, fear, anxiety, recovering the imagination and waking dream (Bion 1970; Ferro 2010) with the aim of trying to work through affective intensities connected to mourning, to the abrupt and brutal loss forced on us by the pandemic. How much of all that we have known and shared in the analytic experiences lived through until today is still standing firm? With B, thanks to our psychic work together, the dramatic event that the psyche had been called upon to live through was trying to become a personal subjective experience for each of us according to our own specific ways of functioning. Alluding to the music of psychoanalytic sounds and using his capacity for "wordplay" – his "verbal scribbling" (Boyer 1999; Ogden 1989) – B introduced a communication able to open up new elaborative possibilities. We discovered together that "the unconscious is alive and capable of development" (Freud 1915, p. 190). We not only had to deal with a knowing that had existed before and been repressed while waiting to reveal itself; more particularly, we were being called upon to cope with a sense that was taking shape in the opening out of possible interpsychic movements which – as happens in poetry, after all – announce "semantic migrations" (Bollas 1989). Such movements of thought and speech may produce new sense through sounds and vocal timbres, but above all, using intuition and imagination, they can make a new possibility resonate in the couple listening to each other. We could call it synaesthetic; the possibility of capturing the whole emotional message that was infusing the atmosphere of the encounter in the remote setting. The original psychic interweaving allowed us a first elaborative form of mourning for the loss we were facing. It was thus an affective experience able to restore the complexity of the many psychic levels that were being brought together at that juncture and in that fragment of analytic exchange, capable of bearing witness to a logic of psychic work as a double, whose deep purpose was to try and keep the shared psychic container alive. In thinking again about this exchange, I recalled Ogden's (1999) reflections in his article "'The Music of What Happens' in Poetry and Psychoanalysis." Quoting Calvino, he states that rhymes between words in poetry have an equivalent in prose narratives: "there are events that rhyme." Expanding a statement like that, we could say that in the experience of psychoanalysis there are conscious and unconscious emotional states of the analyst and the patient that "rhyme" in the sense that they mobilise affects capable of making the two embodied psyches resonate in many ways.

The unconscious often exceeds the forms in which we have learned to understand it using the method that was constructed for grasping its effects. In this painful and traumatic experience that saw us exposed as never before to the condition of impotence, given the sheer range of the difficulties, in that critical moment a thirst for eros and vital force insinuated itself into our unusual encounter. It aroused and continued to sustain the desire to understand where I could establish my internal setting, in listening to the communications coming from new determining conditions.

We should probably look closely again at the specific quality of what is produced by our unconscious, even in such a modified setting. This means trying to deal with the complexity of its derivatives and with the instruments that we have at our disposal for capturing the emerging forms. If we share Freud's assumption that "the unconscious is alive and capable of development," we should then ask ourselves: in what form does it continue to express itself in communication and in listening; from what psychic materials does it get its "voice" and transmit "affective intensities" in such a distinctive setting? The ways in which the devices we adopt produce and organise our psychic life as individuals and in couples continue to enable changes in affective states which pass through our mind and our senses. How does what we hear in words and beyond words reverberate within us and give form to our responses? "It is not so easy to play upon the instrument of the mind," says Freud in a passage from his 1905 essay "On Psychotherapy" (Freud 1905, p. 262). In their heterogeneity not only are the materials that compose our psychic life not easy to play with, they are especially difficult to "listen to" in the countless traces they scatter across the psychic space, prefiguring a sense, representing the past in many ways and at the same time anticipating the future.

Notes

1 The topic of the various listening perspectives in psychoanalysis has been addressed many times as the theoretical constructs of psychoanalysis have evolved. It has pointed up the need to integrate viable theories of listening, which over time have become forms of reciprocal listening, sometimes relegated to verbal productions alone, along very different lines of development on both sides of the ocean. Without going back to the origins of the "third ear" beginning with Reik's (1937) hypotheses, it will be sufficient to illustrate the point by recalling Faimberg's (2005) focus on the idea of "listening to listening." Taking as a starting point the notion of subjective listening and empathic listening, let us also remember all those authors who from Kohut onwards to the post-Kohutian debate, have made listening from the patient's perspective a focal point in theory and practice (I am thinking for example of Schwaber, Fosshage, Aron, Mitchell, and Aktar). To these can be added the theorists of intersubjectivity in their various permutations (for example, Atwood, Stolorow, Brandchaft).

2 Empirical research has highlighted a significant correlation between perception and action: our perception of the world is modelled on action, even when we are not performing a movement, and describes a primal way of knowing the world around us. Our experience of encountering what surrounds us runs in parallel with the experience of ourselves as "potentialities" of bodily action, our perceptual world being an expression of our motor potentialities (Gallese and Sinigaglia 2010). The *mirroring* mechanism expressed by the mirror neurones has mostly been interpreted as linked to the direct and implicit comprehension of other people's behaviour. Nevertheless, we must not forget

that the mirror neurones are also active while we act: thanks to embodied simulation we "resonate" with the moving bodies of others and re simultaneously aware of our own and others' motor possibilities.

3 The description of the processes of subjectivation has been enriched today by a large body of clinical inferences and observational data which converge in delineating an individual that is endowed from the start of life with an innate capacity for connecting to its parents, for perceiving their conscious and unconscious emotional signals and for interpreting their intentions on a level that initially is pre-reflective. The association of the parents' expressive-affective manifestations, especially the facial and vocal, with the child's internal states constitutes the beginning of a distinct emotional category and a first pre-symbolic representation.

4 I emphasise this by noting that in the past decade a series of neuroscientific discoveries have produced interesting new perspectives on unconscious mental functioning and resonated with current conceptual research in psychoanalysis. Indeed, we know today that in the first three years of life childhood experiences are registered in a pre-symbolic code broadly constitutive of a non-repressed unconscious in the implicit memory circuits, mediated on the neural level by the amygdala of the right hemisphere. *So there is a dialectic between brain and experience.* Experience leaves a trace, one that is not only *psychic but also synaptic.*

5 In his concept of *remembered present*, Edelman (1987) demonstrates that perception is associated with memory in the context of a present experience. Thus the past can be constantly re-transcribed in the light of the present. This conception is in tune with the Freudian concept of *Nachträglichkeit* (*après-coup*). The events and experiences of the present contextualise the memory, selecting, assembling, and organising it. As the present experience takes shape it "can alter and re-transcribe previous traces" and thus also the memories of the past. The original memories would be modified and would no longer exist in their previous form (Stern 2010, p. 135). Nevertheless, we cannot fail to take into consideration what clinical experience teaches us, especially with the most serious cases: how difficult some transformations really are; that is to say, how rarely they can create new transcriptions. The role played by traumatic memories appears less in line with the conceptions mentioned previously. I am referring, as I noted a little earlier, to those rigid and pervasive modes of organising experience shown by certain seriously ill patients who tend to select elements of the real according to static invariants. These invariants have the function of maintaining the link between past and present (*identity of perception*) with the aim of guaranteeing continuity, though this is based on poorly adaptive modes of psychic functioning: ties that the past imposes and to which the present must be adapted, or else risk exposure to catastrophic anxieties. Such conditions show that experiences of the past (traces) exist which appear stubbornly resistant to the influence of the present (compulsion to repeat).

6 These hypotheses fit with the recent theories of Karl Friston (2013) which remind us that every living organism must resist the second law of thermodynamics, the spontaneous tendency of every physical system to move towards a state of disorganisation, which can be measured according to degrees of entropy. Friston supposes that biological organisms must protect themselves against high levels of entropy that could cause their death. A high level of entropy signals a great level of disorganisation and may originate in an external source (the environment, for example) or from the organism itself (especially through the natural and spontaneous tendency to disorganisation deriving from the physical and biological properties of matter).

7 I came to know Pirandello's story thanks to a literary encounter with Remo Bodei. This formed the background, perhaps in my preconscious memory, that I was able to draw on in my analytic listening to help me understand a fundamental aspect of my young patient P's psychic functioning which had until then been "mute" in our relationship.

References

Ammaniti M. and Gallese V. (2014). *La nascita dell'intersoggettività. Lo sviluppo del sé tra psico-dinamica e neurobiologia*. Raffaello Cortina, Milan.

Anzieu D. (1985). *The Skin-Ego*. Routledge, Abingdon, 2018.

Anzieu, D. (1996). *Il pensare. Dall'io-pelle all'io-pensante*. Borla, Rome.

Atlas G. and Aron L. (2017). *Dramatic Dialogue: Contemporary Clinical Practice*. Routledge, New York.

Aulagnier P. (1979). *Les destins du plaisir. Aliénation–amour–passion*. PUF, Paris.

Bastianini T (2002). Memorie, modulazione affettiva, azione terapeutica: il contributo delle neuroscienze. Atti XII Congresso Nazionale della Società Psicoanalitica Italiana.

Bastianini T. and Moccia G. (2003). Riflessioni sulle attuali evoluzioni dei concetti di affetto, memoria e azione terapeutica. *Rivista di Psicoanalisi* 49, 3, 529–554.

Bastianini T. (2006). Corpo e psiche sono estesi: il costrutto dell'intersoggettività tra psicoanalisi e neuroscienze. Paper read at an inter-association seminar (AMHP-PIA, AFPP, SIPP, SPI).

Bastianini T. (2009a). Al di qua della simbolizzazione, come «quei frutti che la beccata di un uccello ha fatto maturare troppo in fretta. In Centro Psicoanalitico di Roma, *L'impronta del trauma, sui limiti della simbolizzazione*. Franco Angeli, Milan.

Bastianini T. (2009b). Conoscenza mimetica e comunicazione inconscia. Riflessioni preliminari a un possibile dialogo tra psicoanalisi e neuroscienze. In Moccia G., Solano L. (eds.) *Psicoanalisi e neuroscienze. Risonanze interdisciplinari*. Franco Angeli, Milan.

Bastianini T and Ferruta A. (2018). *La cura psicoanalitica contemporanea. Estensioni della pratica clinica*. Roma, Fioriti.

Bastianini T. (2019). Estensioni della psicoanalisi: eterogeneità dei materiali psichici e pluralità dei costrutti teorici idonei a comprenderli. *Rivista di Psicoanalisi* XV, 4.

Benjamin J. (2017). *Beyond Doer and Done To: Recognition Theory, Intersubjectivity and the Third*. Routledge, New York.

Bion W.R. (1959). Attacks on linking. *The International Journal of Psychoanalysis* 40, 308–315.

Bion W.R. (1962). *Learning from Experience*. Karnac, London.

Bion W.R. (1965). *Transformations*. Karnac, London.

Bion W.R. (1970). *Attention and Interpretation*. Tavistock Publications, London.

Bion, W.R. (1977). *Two Papers: The Grid and Cæsura*. Routledge, Abingdon, 2018.

Bion W.R. (1992). *Cogitations*. Routledge, Abingdon, 2018.

Bion W.R. (1993). A Memoir of the Future. Routledge, London, 2019.

Bion W.R. (2005). The Italian Seminars. In Mawson, C. (ed.) *The Complete Works of W.R. Bion: Vol IX*. Routledge, London, 2005.

Bollas C. (1987). *The Shadow of the Object: Psychoanalysis of the Unthought Known*. Columbia University Press, New York.

Bollas C. (1989). *Forces of Destiny: Psychoanalysis and Human Idiom*. Routledge, New York.

Bollas C. (2007). *The Freudian Moment*. Routledge, New York.

Bollas C. (2008). *The Evocative Object World*. Routledge, New York.

Bollas C. (2009). *The Infinite Question*. Routledge, London.

Botella C. and Botella S. (2001). *La Figurabilité psychique*. Delachaux et Niestlé, Paris. [*The Work of Psychic Figurability*. Routledge, Hove, 2005.]

Bowlby J. (1969). *Attachment and Loss: Volume 1: Attachment*. Basic Books, New York.

Bowlby J. (1973). *Attachment and Loss. Volume 2: Separation: Anxiety and Anger*. Basic Books, New York.

Boyer L.B. (1999). *Countertransference and Regression*. Jason Aronson Inc, Lanham, MA.

Bucci W. (1997). *Psychoanalysis and Cognitive Science*. Guilford, New York.

Cahn R. (2002). *La fin du divan?* Odile Jacob, Paris.

De Toffoli C. (2009). *Il corpo vivente dell'esperienza psicoanalitica. In Transiti Corpo – Mente. L'esperienza della psicoanalisi*. FrancoAngeli, Milan 2014.

Edelman G.M. (1987). *Darwinismo neuronale*. Einaudi, Torino, 1995.

Edelman G.M. (1990). *The Remembered Present: A Biological Theory of Consciousness*. Basic Books, New York.

Faimberg H. (2005). *The Telescoping of Generations: Listening to the Narcissistic Links Between Generations*. Routledge, New York.

Fédida P. (2012). *Aprire la parola. Scritti 1968–2002*. Borla, Rome.

Ferenczi S. (1928). The Elasticity of Psychoanalytic Technique. In *Final Contributions to the Problems and Methods of Psycho-analysis*. Routledge, Abingdon, 2018.

Ferro A. (2010). *Mind Works: Technique and Creativity in Psychoanalysis*. Routledge, London.

Ferruta A. (2015). La clinica psicoanalitica contemporanea. Esperienze psicoanalitiche. *Rivista di Psicoanalisi* 4, 913–929.

Finelli R. (2017). *Il pensiero senza linguaggio. Note sulla rappresentazione in Freud*. Unipress Roma Tre, Rome.

Freud S. (1891). *Zur Auffassung der Aphasien, Eine kritische Studie von Dr. Sigm. Freud, Privatdozent für Neuropathologie an der Universität Wien*. Franz Deuticke, Leipzig-Wien. [*On Aphasia*. International Universities Press, New York, 1953.]

Freud S. (1892–1899). Project for a Scientific Psychology. SE, 1.

Freud S. (1895). *Studies on Hysteria*. SE, 2.

Freud S. (1899, 1900). *The Interpretation of Dreams*. SE, 4–5.

Freud S. (1901). Fragment of an Analysis of a Case of Hysteria (Case study of Dora). SE, 7.

Freud S. (1905). On Psychotherapy. SE, 7.

Freud S. (1909). Notes upon a Case of Obsessional Neurosis (The "Rat Man"). SE, 10.

Freud S. (1912). Recommendations to Physicians Practising Psycho-analysis. SE, 12.

Freud S. (1912–1913). *Totem and Taboo*. SE, 13.

Freud S. (1913) The Claims of Psycho-analysis to Scientific Interest. SE, 13.

Freud S. (1914a). Remembering, Repeating and Working-Through. SE, 12.

Freud S. (1915). The Unconscious. SE, 14.

Freud S. (1922). Two Encyclopaedia Articles: Psycho-Analysis. SE, 18.

Freud S. (1923). The Ego and the Id. SE, 19.

Freud S. (1925a). Negation. SE, 19.

Freud S. (1925b). Inhibitions, Symptoms and Anxiety. SE, 20.

Freud, S. (1927). The Future of an Illusion. SE, 10.

Freud S. (1934–1938). Moses and Monotheism: Three Essays. SE, 23.

Freuta S. (1937). Analysis terminable and interminable. SE, 23.

Freud S. (1938a). An Outline of Psycho-Analysis. SE, 23.

Friston K. (2013). Life as we know it. *Journal of the Royal Society, Interface*, 10.

Fusini N. (2010). *Di vita si muore. Lo spettacolo delle passioni nel teatro di Shakespeare*. Mondadori, Milan.

Gaddini E. (1969). Sulla imitazione. In *Scritti 1953–1985*. Cortina, Milan, 1989.

Gaddini E. (1981). Fantasie difensive precoci e processo psicoanalitico. In *Scritti 1953–1985*. Cortina, Milan, 1989.

Gallese V. and Sinigaglia C. (2010). The Bodily Self as Power for Action. *Neuropsychologia* 49, 9, 2658–2563.

Green A. (1973). *The Fabric of Affect in the Psychoanalytic Discourse*. Routledge, London 1999.

Green A. (1983). *Narcissisme de vie, narcissisme de mort*. Minuit, Paris. [*Life Narcissism, Death Narcissism*. Free Association Books, London, 2001.]

Green A. (1994). *On Private Madness*. Routledge, London, 2018.

Green A. (2002). *Key Ideas for a Contemporary Psychoanalysis: Misrecognition and Recognition of the Unconscious*. Routledge, Hove, 2005.

Green A. (2005). Lezione magistrale del prof. André Green. La mia interpretazione della psicoanalisi. Sogno. Riflessioni della psicoanalisi contemporanea. ETS, Milan.

Green A. (2011). *On Private Madness*. Karnac, London.

Green A. (2012). *La Clinique psychanalytique contemporaine*. Les Éditions d'Ithaque, Paris.

Guerrini Degl'Innocenti B. (2016). Introduzione al seminario "Ripensare l'inconscio".

Jacobs T.J. (1991). *The Use of Self: Countertransference and Communication in the Analytic Situation*. International Universities Press, Madison, TX.

Jacobs T. J. (2007). Review of "The Metapsychology of the Analyst" by Robert Fliess. *Psychoanalytic Quarterly* 76, 3, 715–724.

Kaës R., Faimberg H., Enriquez M. and Baranes J.J. (1993). *Transmission de la vie psychique entre générations*. Dunod, Paris.

Kandel E. (1999) Biology and the Future of Psychoanalysis: A New Intellectual Framework for Psychiatry Revisited. *Am. J. Psychiatry* 156, 505–524.

Kaës R. (2015). *L'estensione della psicoanalisi. Per una metapsicologia di terzo tipo*. Franco Angeli, Milano, 2016.

Klein G. (1976). *Psychoanalytic Theory: An Exploration of Essentials*. International Universities Press, New York.

Klein M. (1932). *The Psycho-Analysis of Children*. Hogarth Press, London.

Kohut H. (1971). *The Analysis of the Self*. Hogarth Press, London.

Krystal H. (1988). *Integration and Self Healing: Affect, Trauma, Alexithymia*. Routledge, New York.

La Scala M. (2017). Percepire, allucinare, immaginare. Il rispecchiamento, il simbolo, il soggetto. *Rivista di Psicoanalisi* 2.

LeDoux J.E. (1996). *The Emotional Brain: The Mysterious Underpinnings of Emotional Life*. Simon & Schuster, New York.

Loewald H. (1980). *Papers on Psychoanalysis*. Yale University Press, New Haven and London.

Lyons-Ruth K. (1998). Implicit Relational Knowing: Its Role in Development and Psychoanalytic Treatment. *Infant Mental Health Journal* 19, 3, 282–289.

Lyons-Ruth K. (2003). Dissociation and the Parent Infant Dialogue: A Longitudinal Perspective from Attachment Research. *Journal of the American Psychoanalytic Association* 51, 833–914.

Matthis I. (2000). Sketch for a Metapsychology of Affect. *International Journal of Psychoanalysis* 81, 215–227.

Merleau-Ponty M. (1945). *Phenomenology of Perception*. Routledge, Abingdon, 2012.

Merleau-Ponty, M. (1953). Les Sciences de l'homme et la phénoménologie. Centre de Documentation Universitaire, Paris.

Merleau-Ponty M. (1964). *Le Visible et l'invisible*. Gallimard, Paris.

Milner M. (1955). The Role of Illusion in Symbol Formation. In Gosso S. (ed) *Psychoanalysis and Art. Kleinian Perspectives*. Routledge, London.

Modell A.H. (1993). *The Private Self*. Harvard University Press, Boston MA.

Modell A. H. (2009). Metaphor—The Bridge between Feelings and Knowledge. *Psychoanalytic Inquiry* 29, 1, 6–11.

Nissim Momigliano L. (1984). "Due persone che parlano in una stanza" (Una ricerca sul dialogo analitico). *Rivista di Psicoanalisi* 30, 1, 1–17.

Ogden T. (1989). *The Primitive Edge of Experience*. Routledge, New York.

Ogden T. (1999). "The Music of What Happens" in Poetry and Psychoanalysis. *International Journal of Psychoanalysis* 80, 979–994.

Ogden T. (2000). Foreword. In Meares R. (ed.) *Intimacy and Alienation: Memory, Trauma and Personal Being*. Routledge, Abingdon.

Ogden T. (2005). *This Art of Psychoanalysis: Dreaming Undreamt Dreams and Interrupted Cries*. Routledge, New York.

Ogden T. H. (2016). *Reclaiming Unlived Life: Experiences in Psychoanalysis*. Routledge, London.

Panksepp J. (2012). *The Archaeology of Mind: Neuroevolutionary Origins of Human Emotions*. Norton, New York.

Pessoa F. (2016). "This." In *Poeti di Lisbona*. Artes Grafica, Lisbon, Portugal.

Putnam F. (1997). *Dissociation in Children and Adolescents: A Developmental Perspective*. Guilford Press, New York.

Reik T. (1937). *Surprise and the Psycho-Analyst: On the Conjecture and Comprehension of Unconscious Process*. Dutton and Company, New York.

Ricœur P. (2020). *Attorno alla psicoanalisi*. Barale F. (ed.). Jaca Book, Milan.

Riolo F. (1978). L'"agire" come linguaggio e rappresentazione. *Rivista di Psicoanalisi* 3.

Roussillon R. (2002). Ombre et transformation de l'objet. *Revue française de psychanalyse* 66, 1825–1835.

Roussillon R. (2006). Pluralité de l'appropriation subjective. In Richard F. and Wainrib S. (eds.) *La subjectivation*. Dunod, Paris.

Roussillon R. (2018). Paradigmi per un'estensione della pratica psicoanalitica. In Bastianini T. and Ferruta A. (eds.) *La cura psicoanalitica contemporanea*. Giovanni Fioriti editore, Rome.

Sapisochin G. (2013). Second Thoughts on Agieren: Listening to the Enacted. International *Journal of Psychoanalysis* 94, 967–991.

Searles H. (1979). *Countertransference and Related Subjects: Selected Papers*. International Universities Press, Madison, TX.

Steiner J. (1993). *Psychic Retreats: Pathological Organizations in Psychotic, Neurotic and Borderline*. Routledge, New York.

Stern D. (1985). *The Interpersonal World of the Infant*. Basic Books, New York.

Stern D. (2004). *The Present Moment in Psychotherapy and Everyday Life*. Norton, New York.

Stern D. (2010). *Forms of Vitality: Exploring Dynamic Experience in Psychology, the Arts, Psychotherapy, and Development*. OUP, Oxford.

Thelen E. and Smith L. (1994). *A Dynamic Systems Approach to the Development of Cognition and Action*. MIT Press, Cambridge, MA.

Tronick E. (1998). Dyadically Expanded States of Consciousness and the Process of Therapeutic Change. *Infant Mental Health Journal* 19, 290–299.

Turillazzi Manfredi S. and Pazzagli A. (1986). Acting-out. *Rivista di Psicoanalisi*, 30, 93–105.

Van der Kolk B. (2014). *The Body Keeps the Score: Brain, Mind, and Body in the Healing of Trauma*. Penguin, New York.

Varela (1991). Il corpo come macchina ontologica. In Preta L. (ed.) *Che cos'è la conoscenza*. Laterza, Bari, 43–52.

Williams R. (ed.) (2009). *Trauma e relazioni. Le prospettive scientifiche e cliniche contemporanee*. Raffaello Cortina, Milan.

Winnicott D. W. (1941). The Observation of Infants in a Set Situation. *The International Journal of Psycho Analysis* 22, 229–249.

Winnicott D.W. (1945). Primitive Emotional Development. In *Collected Papers: Through Paediatrics to Psycho-Analysis*. Tavistock, London, 1958, 145–156.

Winnicott D.W. (1948). Reparation in Respect of Mother's Organised Defence Against Depression. In *Collected Papers: Through Paediatrics to Psycho-Analysis*. Tavistock, London, 1958, 91–100.

Winnicott D.W. (1949). Mind and its Relation to the Psyche-Soma. In *Collected Papers: Through Paediatrics to Psycho-Analysis*. Tavistock, London, 1958, 243–255.

Winnicott D.W. (1956). Primary Maternal Preoccupation. In *Collected Papers: Through Paediatrics to Psycho-Analysis*. Tavistock, London, 1958, 300–306.

Winnicott D.W. (1965). *The Family and Individual Development*. Tavistock, London.

Winnicott D.W. (1971). *Playing and Reality*. Tavistock Publications, London.

Winnicott D.W. (1974). Editorial Note. Fear of Breakdown. *International Review of Psychoanalysis* 1, 103–107.

Winnicott D.W. (1986). *Holding and Interpretation*. International Psychoanalytic Library, London.

Chapter 2

Embodied unconsciouses

In the beginning was action

Benedetta Guerrini Degl'Innocenti

What is the unconscious? How could we, psychoanalysts of the third millennium, answer this question 120 years after the publication of the "Egyptian dream book" (Freud 1887–1904)? Though we experience it directly every day, it is as if the unconscious is an unstable material, invisible by its very nature, which, like molecular matter, needs an ever more refined technique if we are to discover the large amount that we still do not know. And the more we refine our instruments, the more we develop our theories, and the more we discover new multiform and powerful manifestations of the unconscious.

Having advanced through the territory of its first formidable explorations, psychoanalysis has ventured beyond the Pillars of Hercules of its own initial theoretical capability. And there it has encountered memories that could not be remembered, traumas that could not be put into words, and psychic functionings so extreme as to pose a powerful challenge to the analytic device. In the effort to add ever more precise detail to the quality of the psychoanalytic instrument, without which there can be neither knowledge nor cure, but at the same time not accepting the abandonment of humanity to their limitations, to a destiny of suffering, ignorance, and conformism, the extension of psychoanalytic clinical practice has steadily widened the field of what the psychic is. Analysts have thus found themselves confronted with a vast area of manifestations that do not yet have words (sensory traces, somatic manifestations, muscular movements, actions) but may nevertheless have a powerful communicative value: actions, or rather enactments, that may represent an extreme attempt to give form to the formless in situations where the capacity for representation is damaged. The concept of action, an inescapable condition of our very being in the world, has gone through a long and troubled conceptual trajectory in psychoanalysis. Ruggiero (2017) rightly points out how the concept of action has in a certain sense encountered the same fate as the countertransference: from being an element talked about only *inter nos*, a testimony of the analyst's existence as a person, as dangerous as it is irrepressible, and hence an attack on the myth of the analyst as pure "analysing function," to an element that may contain transformative features capable of activating the analytic process, especially in those situations where figurability, as the Botellas call it, must be considered as an outcome of communication and not yet an instrument available to the analytic process.

DOI: 10.4324/9781003544647-2

As Eugenio Gaddini (1984) wrote 40 years ago, psychoanalysts have spent more than a century investigating the pathology of mental functioning and, thereby, natural mental functioning. Psychoanalysis, born from the genius of one man based on the observation and treatment of neurotic pathologies, has developed an extraordinary body of theory in a hundred years, and psychoanalysts have progressively refined their knowledge, diagnostic ability, and technique, and consequently widened the scope for therapeutic intervention. It is taken for granted that psychoanalysts today find themselves performing their function even with patients who have for a long time been considered inaccessible to psychoanalytic therapy. On the other hand, looking at fundamental psychic phenomena and processes such as the limitations of consciousness, the defences, resistances to treatment, the transference and countertransference in a more exhaustive way than any other theory of the mind – phenomena that must necessarily be integrated in the understanding of clinical work if we want to offer a suitable and effective psychological treatment – psychoanalysis could not hold back from the need to regain the space that it can and must occupy in the field of disciplines concerned with the mind.

Indeed, psychoanalysis is more and more often asked to address clinical situations that show heterogeneous characteristics from the viewpoint of psychopathological phenomenology, but represent an interesting stimulus for theory and a fertile testing ground for the analytic device. I am referring in particular to patients who, in their clinical presentation and psychic functioning, do not seem to fit into the traditional neurotic pathologies, without, however, corresponding to the often stereotypical fixity of the psychotic scenarios. They are forms that can be characterised by a pervasive lack of structure and organisation and by an almost total inability to construct representations of internal states so that they can be put into words. The affective states, as they are manifested in the session, emerge as neither integrated nor structured, in most cases lacking representational contents and lived as predominantly sensory experiences, indistinct and often menacing in the disorganising effect they seem to bring with them: a *feeling of affective overflow* that seems to suffocate the psyche (Green 1975). In contact with these patients, one is struck by the poverty of their fantasy life, as if the psyche were constantly stuck in the actual (Green 2002): an actual that never manages to become familiar and predictable because it is instead rendered disturbing by the impossibility of building it a psychic figurability that could be inserted into a personal narrative. The very nature of the identificatory and subjectivating processes is powerfully influenced by this deficient representational function: identification ends up being more or less kaleidoscopic and the processes of subjectivation are made impossible by the persistence of unintegrated states of the self that are aggregated sensorially around affective nuclei which, being unable to attain the sphere of representation, cannot be integrated or used to construct the sense of self.

They are people who in some respects recall the "heterogeneous patients" that Danielle Quinodoz talks about, patients who seem to ask for help because they are suffering excessively from their heterogeneity, who "feel anxiety because they have not been able to integrate the different aspects of *themselves* and are afraid they will not be capable of maintaining their sense of internal unity" and often express more or less implicitly or directly "the anxiety of going mad" (Quinodoz 2005).

Another pervasive characteristic of these patients is *enactment*: by this intentionally ambiguous term I mean to indicate a broad spectrum of actions without a single psychic meaning. Alongside the commonest and most frequently described *moves into action* – expressions of the more classic motility of the reflexive, direct, and automatic type, a path of discharge operated by the primary process (Freud 1899) – other forms may coexist: actions that seem to want to speak, that seem to be searching for someone who knows how to read their communicative valence, their effort to give form to the formless.

So my reflections in this section of the book aim to integrate themes that have interested me for a long time, such as the varied, complex, and unavoidable relations between action and representation: tracing the path from the most overtly evacuative action to the "dramatised" action aimed at representation and located in a scenic space. An acting, as Riolo (1978) writes, "endowed with meaning and communicative value, through which the world of the internal objects is externalised and re-presented, sometimes in the consulting room, sometimes outside it, but in any case *inside* the analytic relationship," so that it can reveal its communicative impulse by means of that powerful relational device that is the transference-countertransference relationship.

In Bion's words:

> If I cannot make myself clear verbally, then I might fall back on actions, which speak louder than words. If I were a baby I could try screaming. If my mother was unable to understand that, I might become so frightened by the noise that I fell silent, then nobody, not even I, could hear my screams. I might have to find actions instead. If I grew up and found an analyst, I might try acting-out.
>
> (Bion 1973, p. 48)

Looking at these actions that speak louder than words, I will trace their pathways, motivations, and transformative possibilities in the encounter with the mind of the analyst.

Daniel and the edge of chaos

"I'm here because a bomb has exploded inside me," he tells me during our first conversations. And as he goes into detail about the tortured romantic relationship that has prompted him to seek help, he shows an increasing puzzlement about the meaning he should attribute to the events and his partner's motivations, and to their context, and his speech is impregnated with an anxious state of alarm, strangeness, and a pervasive sense of impotence and rage.

Initially all attempts on my part to understand any of this fail miserably, and the only result is to immerse me in the same indistinct magma where he is floundering. I come out of the first meetings with him feeling that I have understood nothing and simultaneously committed to trying to reconstruct what *really* happened in a way that seems a bit demented at the time but also fundamental, as if something essential for psychic survival revolved around the ascertaining of the truth.

After several sessions have been spent struggling against the frightening confusion that seems to be devastating his mind, I find myself thinking about the game in the weekly puzzle magazine where you have to identify some bizarre objects contained in an ordinary scene, densely packed with details, people, and things. I think that perhaps the problem does not consist of identifying the characteristics of the object (*the girlfriend* or *the incident*), but in the disorganising and confusing activity of the attempt to *understand*. Trying to put together an intervention that might include both the feeling of urgency about finding out the truth and the growing feeling of confusion that derives from it, I tell him that it seems to me as if the attempt to understand is creating a frightening confusion in his head: confusion about the events and their consequences, but also about the emotions deriving from it, and even confusion about who did or thought what. The intervention seems to stop him in his tracks, and he says that confusion is actually a problem he has always struggled with and that sometimes he suspects it might be really serious because his mind "wanders in a way you just wouldn't believe."

The day after: Looking himself in the face so as not to lose himself

The first year of work with Daniel has really been like picking one's way through the site of a nuclear explosion: his speech constantly breaks down and turns into a sort of expulsion of disconnected mental bits and pieces containing stubs of fact, ambiguous hints, sketches of thought with no clear origin. Contact with him had strong connotations of "fragmentation" and "confusion," both about himself (from losing things to having no idea what he did a moment before; from not knowing how to do even the most banal things to having no clear image of himself) and about other people. For him, *other people* seem to be indecipherable, mysterious objects because he appears unable to contain them as objects endowed with their own subjectivity except via a few stereotyped fragments of *inter-actions*.

At the start it is even difficult to transcribe sessions. Following the thread of his thoughts is only possible by immersing oneself in the atmosphere of *the day after*[1] that he seems to be suspended in: traumatic, confused, and dissociated. Much of his mental activity seems to be governed by the primary process: he cannot bear gratification to be deferred, and he has no consideration for the consequences of his actions. His reasoning often lacks a logical structure and a careful testing of reality which he might be able to translate into the making of plans and a full awareness of the relationship between means and ends. His mind seems to operate not on the basis of rational and realistic principles but on a basis of insignificant or stereotyped similarities: what Freud calls *superficial association*, which often relies on an echo of assonances, sometimes taking concepts on board purely because of a temporal coincidence, with no close relationship in their meaning.

At the same time, in terms of object-representation, Daniel seems to be stuck in a very early phase of development: a stage that we could call *sensorimotor*, in which the object is invested exclusively at the moment when it gratifies the need, but remains relatively undifferentiated and internally re-presented almost entirely by its capacity to provide gratification. There is scant awareness of the other, who never appears in his mind completely separate from the context of experience; as if the object were experienced on the basis of its activities and its image were nothing but an extrapolation of patterns of action (like the stereotyped descriptions of his women, always using the same examples with which he reports sequences of actions or rigid verbal exchanges that are made incomprehensible by the absence of a general context and an adequate level of abstraction). The consequent undifferentiation in representing the object is inextricably connected to an insufficient differentiation between self and object, to the extent of inducing experiences of deep and disorganising *con-fusion*, as in the encounter with *the foreign girl* (as he called her) which had resulted in his decision to contact me.

During the first year, the sessions were often total immersions in his confusion: whole sessions from which I emerged feeling as if I'd been on a motorbike going at 200 kmph in fog, hardly able to see anything clearly, using most of my mental energy to *stay on the saddle* and not plunge into the chaos where he was. His mind's functioning appeared to be mostly sensory and strongly impregnated with turbulence, confusion, and asymbolic excitation, as if his psychic survival were only guaranteed by constant rapid movement, to avoid being knocked over by contact with the other's mind, which is something mysterious and incomprehensible, oppressive and disorganising.

For the whole of the first year, I simply listened and, where the confused flow of his thoughts allowed an opening, added a stitch or two to his unseamed thinking to keep it together while we waited for him to glimpse the overall fabric. Much of the analytic process, at least where it was possible to have one, took place in my mind, balancing like a tightrope walker between negative capability and the wait for a *scrap of meaning* (Ferro 2010).

After the first year, spent alternating between phases when speech was possible and others that were extremely confused, it gradually occurred to me that if I modified the way our meetings were set up it might help the analytic apparatus to realise its potential more fully: I am thinking of increasing the number of sessions and suggesting that Daniel use the couch. I am prompted to do this by the fact that he has started dreaming, though without any associations unless I specifically ask for them, and also by the need I feel more and more strongly to add nuance to my concrete presence; partly to reduce the *inter-action*, beginning with his tendency to *make me do* things, and partly in order maintain the privacy that is necessary if we are to be mutually receptive, in the best way possible, to unconscious communications. I realise that the work we are doing is actually creating a potential space for working-through when he is the one who suggests the third session.

Once we changed the setting it slowly became possible to transform the apparently senseless chaos of his life – a chaos with no solution, made of things and actions rather than relationships and emotional states – into a mode of mental functioning we could try and think about. The objects that he flung around the consulting room every time he arrived, and which sometimes ended up being lost somewhere, began to be gathered into a bag large enough to contain his things, and full of pockets where he could find them again. He moved from keeping his phone on and answering it every time it rang, to checking whether the call was important enough to need answering, and then to keeping it silent and hardly ever answering it. It slowly became possible for him to stay silent, which I registered in the countertransference as his having acquired the ability *to be alone in the presence of the other person*; never for very long and often only after a highly intense exchange in which I offered him an integration of scattered fragments that had accumulated to a certain point in my mind.

Giving form to the object

The transference relationship, like Daniel's identity, begins to crystalise around a superficial dependence on my opinions, which are always solicited by direct questions or indirect hints. He also adapts well to the setting, and is almost always punctual. Above all, he never gets the day or time of his session wrong, which is quite extraordinary given the apparent disorganisation and confusion of his daily life. I feel that for him I am a powerful, omniscient object with whom to develop a relationship of "parental" dependency: that is, expecting me to do things for him, as his parents did, giving him the answers that could diminish his confusion. Sometimes he abruptly stands up and goes over to his briefcase, asking if I could take a quick look at something he has to deliver, if I could tell him whether it is suitable because he has no idea, suddenly finding a need in his head that the object should satisfy straightaway.

He often asks me direct questions about what I think he should do or say, or else he makes a statement and immediately follows it with, "Or not?"

At the same time, also in the transference, a markedly split object relationship has emerged in which the need for the object is immediately fraught with rage and anxiety, and his confusion increasingly takes on the characteristics of a defence: a defence against the anxiety of being invaded by the object, by its demands, expectations, and needs, and at the same time a defence against the rage that could be unleashed to attack the object, destroying it. In other words, on the couch he is very polite, friendly, and engaged, then he crushes my hand when we say goodbye at the door. Splitting, idealisation, and projection are the predominant defensive strategies and, as a result, self and object are poorly differentiated.

For example, he might happen to lie down and say, "Listen … on Friday or Saturday I texted to ask if we were going to see each other on Monday …" And for a fraction of a second I'm confused and wonder what text he's talking about; did he want another session on Monday? Then I realise that, without naming her, he is talking about the *foreign girl* he usually sees on Mondays.

To me, the "misunderstanding" that begins this exchange seems suggestive of an identification/counter-identification in which he relates to me in the same way as he relates to all his women: not as subjects external to him, with whom to hold a dialogue and to whom he should therefore make himself comprehensible, but as narcissistically invested internal objects lacking a life and subjectivity of their own. He is not speaking to me but relating to the internal object-analyst, an omniscient object who knows without any need for him to bother with explanations. But she is a "non-subjectivated" object so he can avoid being persecuted by her; an object *not-other-than-himself*, for whom he has no responsibility, not even the need to make himself understood.

I think this short-circuiting of identification/counter-identification is also evidence of the extremely vague self–other boundaries that characterise him, as is the lack of an ability to distinguish one person from another, which means that all other people are part of groups (the women he is with, his friends – female or male – the colleagues in his department, etc.) in which there is little differentiation between individuals. But at the same time, as groups, they seem to be characterised in a repetitive, hyper-simplified and almost caricatured way. The whole effort of this analysis has been to maintain a sort of "stable instability": patient and analyst inextricably linked, contained in a single dynamic process which oscillates between the need for some kind of order and the irresistible urge towards chaos, between a neediness that cannot desire and a hungry dependency that does not admit the other's subjectivity.

Daniel is a patient who enables us to grasp highly complex countertransferential situations which put us in contact with a turbulent self, endlessly on a knife edge: a self that seems to live constantly "on the brink" of some action, always motivated by contingent micro-necessities which cannot be deferred and lack real psychic intentionality. Over time I found myself thinking about Daniel's modes of being in the world as *representations in action*. This expression, used by Sidney Blatt (1974) with reference to pre-operational modes of representation linked to the sensorimotor stages as conceived by Piaget (Piaget and Inhelder 1966), seemed to capture his way of *being in action*, which is a primitive, sensory, asymbolic form of representation.

In more specifically psychoanalytic terms, these particular representations can be considered as representations of the primary process (Schafer 1968), characterised by carelessness, instability, spatial indeterminacy, lack of reflectiveness, and scant differentiation between self and not-self. As Blatt (1974) emphasises, at an early sensorimotor stage representations are based on sequences of actions: the relational modes are immediate and entail physical reflex reactions that may be as motoric as they are affective, and are often directed to the satisfaction of biological needs.

Even if there is some awareness of the object, this is never completely separate from the context of experience and the event currently in progress.

At this level the object is experienced in terms of its activities, its representation being an extrapolation of the action pattern. The object is recognised and valued only in the specific limited context of need gratification, and it has little meaning or existence beyond providing comfort and alleviating pain.

(Blatt 1974, p. 143)

This particular mode began to be thinkable following some small attempts on my part to offer Daniel metaphors that might give his *being in things* a form that was not merely enacted. When, for example, the focus was on his chronic difficulty in reconstructing what had led him to sleep with one of those numerous women, it did not seem possible for him to recognise either the prompting of a desire or any intentionality, at least a conscious one. I had a mental impression like a kind of inescapable atmospheric event, an almost sensory reverie that I often experienced during his laborious and unproductive attempts to find a psychic explanation for these events ("I left work, called in on her, we went to bed" or "I did it ... we were there, it happened") so I put this impression to use and at a certain point I commented, "It rained!"

Thanks to this first sketchy figurability (Botella and Botella 2001) evoked by "a temporary and transitory condition of companionable, cooperative fusion" (Bolognini 2008, p. 69) and strongly coloured by the pre-representational sensoriality that was characteristic of Daniel, it was possible for him to start thinking about his difficulty in giving a personal sense to the relationship with the other and to the events of his life. My "it rained!" may be read as a preliminary unsaturated psychic form, open to various meanings and developments: something that does not provide a ready-made meaning but contains a "generative potential for sense" (Di Benedetto 2000). Something that starts to *put into-form* without yet *giving a form*.

It rained became the expression Daniel learned to use whenever he had to describe an action of his that apparently made no personal or relational sense. This small shared metaphor, as it became in our private lexicon, allowed us slowly to grasp how this *lack of sense* could be linked to his parents' failure to acknowledge his subjectivity and intentionality by acting for him whenever there was a decision to be made.

I think it was also thanks to this that, in the next few sessions, Daniel was able to gain access to one of the rare memories from his childhood, an extremely painful memory of his father saying to him when he was very young, "It's no use wondering what you've got in your brain, because there isn't anything in your brain!"

At the start of the fourth year a new object appears in his life: Tina, a woman of his own age (like the analyst) whom he had met previously and who suddenly enters his visual field and strikes him not because of a series of stereotyped and superficial characteristics but because of the warm affectivity she displays, the gentleness with which she is able to accept him, and her ability to leave him alone when he starts to get restive. In a very intense session he tells me that the night before, while they were awake, he said to her, "I'd like to come inside you." She answered, "Do." He tells me that she hadn't understood: "I meant just like a child

…" I say that this may be exactly what he means every time he asks me, insistently and a bit anxiously, if I have understood: he is wondering if I can *understand*, beyond the words, something that comes *before words*; a desire to feel he is so inside me that he doesn't have to *explain*, but just *feel together*. He is asking me if I can understand with *his head*.

A deep relationship is being formed with Tina in which for the first time he feels understood and accepted, and this enables him to transform *acting to keep himself together* into *doing things together*, including the experience of caregiving when his girlfriend develops an orthopaedic problem which for over a year makes it hard for her to be independent, until she has an operation.

For many years the *foreign girl* continues to be a turbulent but essential presence, the outcome of a split that seems not to have been integrated, charged with such a potent and unrepresentable excitation that it can only be compulsively acted in an always equal repetition.

During the fifth year of analysis Daniel begins to find small but significant images which seem to transform the *foreign girl* from a picture in an album, two-dimensional and without a life of her own, into an internal object endowed with a great and highly dangerous power of attraction, but one that it is possible to start thinking about. In describing her, he tells me she is

> "like a background noise: sometimes she makes a huge racket, sometimes not so much. Being with her is like being in a big noisy room: you don't know which direction you're going in and you don't know what you're looking for".

Shortly before he manages to leave her for good, an action and its symbolic equivalent appear for the first time in the same sentence: "Now I'd really like to get rid of her, from my home, but especially from inside me." And a little later, talking about his home, he adds, "I need to sort things out there, so I can sort things out inside myself."

Analytic device and symbolic transformation: Giving form to the formless

Analysis with patients like Daniel confronts the analyst with a vast area of manifestations *that do not yet have words* but, at the same time, may have a potent communicative valence. In this particular type of action, which I would call *representations in action*, the function of transforming reality, intrinsic in the act, and from which its communicative function derives, does not disappear (as it does in exclusively expulsive acting) if it can meet the analyst's mind in the transferential–countertransferential scene. My hypothesis is that *enactments* are an extreme attempt to give form to the formless in situations where the capacity for representation is damaged; this damage stops the transformation of emotions, and so they invade the psyche in their most raw state, disorganising any possibility of thought. In these cases, the outward discharge is not an attempt to expel a molesting or painful thought, but the consequence of the impossibility of producing it. So the *enactment* simultaneously appears to be a *character in search of an author* and a way of avoiding the *psychic constipation* produced by the impossibility of metabolising the raw sensory experience.

Taking into account the distinctive functioning of Daniel's mind, I think I can say that the analytic device consisting of the setting and the analytic function of the analyst's mind, maintaining a certain degree of *stable instability*, was able to contain both Daniel and his internal objects, which initially were dispersed *in suspension*, then slowly in a more *aggregated* state. The dependable constancy of the setting, vitally dynamic and not repetitively stereotyped, functioned at first as a container of part-objects – pallid two-dimensional forms *in action* – and then slowly catalysed the generative power of the transference–countertransference relationship which enabled us to start transforming what seemed to be mere *actions in themselves* into *representations of the Self* and of the other.

During the analysis with Daniel I tried to use my hearing as the *receiver* described by Freud; listening attentively to whatever presents itself, whether a sound, a noise, or an uproar, until something unexpectedly starts to come forward: an idea, image or word, Freud's *Einfall* (a mental content emerging into consciousness without, so to speak, being invited) that may be able to give form to the formless. This complex psychic movement, which Bollas calls *countertransference dreaming* (Bollas 1995, p. 12) and which is simply the analyst's partly conscious, partly unconscious response to contact with the patient's mind, can transform action into thought and emptiness into representation. In other words, that process, inhibited and inaccessible in the patient's mind, can be set in motion – by proxy, as it were – in the mind of the analyst.

Giving psychic form to the beginnings of experience: From action to representation

From the start, the subject's encounter with the world and the objects contained in it is an exciting and terrible experience. From the moment of birth the infant is exposed to a constant, relentless experience made of innumerable sensory contacts with unknown objects and violent sensations, states alternating with each other that can neither be controlled nor, at the time, comprehended.

The element that the infant has innately available for sketching out a first discrimination relates to the sensation of pleasure or unpleasure that contact with the object evokes sensorially in the infant himself. But to give psychic form to the first experience and regulate its intensity, and then to achieve a distinction between me and not-me, the infant needs another mind, a *Nebenmensch*, as Freud called that *nearest human being* who can fulfil the original function of the other (Freud 1895).

The human mind's innate urge to give psychic form to experience with the world thus depends, in large part, on the presence of the other, and from the beginning the achievement of the human process of subjectivation assumes a cultural valence based on the relational, affective, and cognitive context that makes it possible

(Giaconia et al. 2008): this primary context is the apparatus of "the care it receives from its mother," without which, says Freud (1911, p. 219n), the infant "organisation could not maintain itself alive for the shortest time."

If we look at the dawn of life we see how the infant has a sensory, pre-representational affectivity (Racalbuto 1994), a "psychosomatic functioning": a sort of primal infantile skill that makes continuity possible, the *going on being* that Winnicott (1965) talks about, faced with the states of incessant and tumultuous psychophysical discontinuity that the child runs into. In this primeval phase of psychic life, any perturbation of physiological homoeostasis results for the child in a reaction that it expresses as immediate and automatic motor actions, such as crying, kicking, or waving its arms: a *body-mind* in action with the aim of re-establishing the lost homoeostatic equilibrium. These actions of response, which we could call primordial defensive modes of the not yet integrated or subjectivated body-ego, need a maternal mind that transforms them from bodily experiences into affective states, into thoughts that can be thought, put into words, and shared.

Out of the initially diffuse, then gradually more organised dust cloud of innumerable contacts that the baby has every day with its mother – the mother who feeds it, talks to it, scolds it, and so on – based on the subjective experiences in the interaction with her, the baby gradually creates a representation of the mother which moves beyond contingent/present experience: that is, an organisation is created, a schema or a set of rules that organise the data of subjective experience (Sandler and Rosenblatt 1962).

As time goes by, the representations that the baby creates of its own objects, of itself, and its body become stable. And it is from that moment onwards that the representations acquire the anticipatory function which allows the child to read reality and make predictions. The presence of an external object is therefore a foundational condition for constructing the ability to represent.

In the beginning was action

From the outset, from the first sight of everything in the shared space, the encounter with the other is permeated by actions or their effects. As Freud (1925) maintains, our psychic life, the *primum movens* of our knowledge of the world and of ourselves, is born from a first action: putting in – spitting out; and this first *doing* is the origin of the distinction between inside and outside, between me and not-me, between the Self and the other. And in one part of itself, the whole personality always remains physical, rooted in action (Ambrosiano 2009).

In normal development the bodily Self and the psychological Self form the sense of Self together: the bodily Self is the founding nucleus, the container, of the psychological Self (Freud 1923). As I said in the previous chapter, sensations and bodily experiences play an essential role in development and any perturbation of the physiological homoeostasis results for the infant in a reaction expressed, as we said earlier, in the form of immediate and automatic motor actions such as yelling, kicking, or waving the arms. "The power of movement," writes Freud in Chapter

VI of the *Traumdeutung*, "which is in the first instance a means of bringing about internal alterations in its body, is at its disposal as the path to discharge" (Freud 1899, p. 598).

For the child, these response actions, which act as attempts to achieve a homoeostatic equilibrium between the internal state and the external object, can gradually acquire an *iconic* function (Campbell and Enckell 2005) thereby becoming primitive representations or, paraphrasing Freud, *presentations of experience*. Since the child's reactions happen within the relationship with the caregiving figure, these motoric schemata, modulated or rigidified by the quality of the affects evoked in the exchange, are thus progressively integrated in primary object relations.

In normal development certain gestures or particular sequences deriving from the daily mother–child interactions can express a specific experience without the child necessarily being aware of it. Like Campbell and Enckell, I believe these behavioural acts mirror the constituting of *primordial representations* of how the other is experienced: in other words, a motor act becomes the primordial presentation of a mental experience in which the object (in this case, the experience) and the representation are identical. The work of progressively constructing representational scenarios is thus developed from the starting point of a pre- or proto-representation of action or movement with *neither object nor subject* (Roussillon 2015), a representation on the way to becoming a narrative form of *being in relation to*, the way the subject narrates their experience in the primary encounter with the object.

Over the course of our existence, when we feel a desire we activate in ourselves the (usually unconscious) fantasy of a specific inter-action that has been experienced in the past as gratifying (or a set of such inter-actions) and the roles played in it by the characters involved (Filippini and Zavattini 1999). In this connection, quoting Freud, Sandler (1990) cites the concept of *identity of perception*, maintaining that over the course of their whole existence, the individual seeks the same type of interaction that was experienced as gratifying in the past (although we should add that these can be pathological).

In order to achieve this *identity of perception* – that is, the same type of gratification of desire that was obtained in the past – the individual may follow various paths. The most common consists in acting in such a way as to provoke the desired response in the other, thereby realising the gratifying fantasy. If, instead of resorting to sublimation, which results in a creative and socially acceptable activity, the subject seeks to gratify the desire on the basis of *identity of perception* – essentially, if they seek a gratification constructed on the model of what they experienced in pathogenic contexts in the past – then they deploy pathological behaviours aimed at reproducing pathogenic relationships.

Reproduction is in itself an elaborate form of repetition and, I would like to add, more than this, a further form of action. So action is everywhere, even if it manifests itself in a variety of forms: muscular, when acting is directed outwards; neuroendocrinal when the acting happens in the body; virtual and experiential when it is expressed in thoughts and words. The first two forms are those that need "reproduction in the psychical field" (Freud 1914, p. 153) through a more radical transformation than is needed when well-formulated thoughts momentarily evade awareness, so that their reproduction simply involves turning the beam of consciousness onto them (Scarfone 2013).

The work of the psyche-soma: From intercorporeality to communication in speech

It is undeniable that, for most of its history, human language has been spoken language. This seems to suggest that language evolved primarily to provide the individual with a powerful and flexible cognitive instrument for sharing, communicating, and exchanging knowledge (see Tomasello et al. 2005). Although opinion in this field is not unanimous, biologists and neuroscientists agree on the fact that our language is the evolution of other, probably poorer, language forms that were still capable of quite complex forms of communication.

One of the hypotheses in the field maintains that our language is the final stage of evolution from a gestural language. As Ludwig Wittgenstein said: "What we call meaning must be connected with the primitive language of gestures" (Wittgenstein 1953). According to this hypothesis, the human species that acquired the Broca and Wernicke areas developed a complex gestural language also enriched by sounds. When the phonatory apparatus later evolved in *Homo sapiens*, and with it the possibility of articulating numerous complex sounds, speech gained the upper hand without, however, completely ousting gestures from communication between individuals. This hypothesis is validated by the fact that in our brain the language and motor control areas are largely the same. Tomasello maintains that linguistic communication is founded, to a greater extent than it may at first seem, on uncoded communication and on other forms of "mental attunement" (Tomasello 2008, p. 59). The linguistic code would rest on a non-linguistic infrastructure of intentional comprehension and on a common conceptual terrain, whose role would in fact be primarily logical (Wittgenstein 1953). In other words, the foundations of human communication would rest on a non-conventionalised and uncoded communication such as human beings' natural gestures: simple gestures like pointing and pantomiming that are used to communicate in powerful and species-specific ways. Viewed in terms of their relational function – that is, the way they are used to communicate – humans use gestures to:

- Direct a recipient's attention in space towards something in the immediate perceptual environment (*deictic* use), the pointing which the child develops at around 9–12 months;
- Direct the recipient's imagination towards something that is usually not found in the immediate perceptual environment, behaviourally simulating an action, a relationship, or an object (*iconic* use).

(Tomasello 2008)

The explanation of why human beings are capable of communicating with each other in a highly complex manner with such simple gestures is that they cooperate in species-specific ways that entail processes of shared intentionality (Tomasello 2008). According to some philosophers of action (Gilbert 1989), shared intentionality refers to behavioural phenomena that are both intentional and irreducibly social in the sense that the agent of the intentions and actions is the plural subject "we." And according to Tomasello (2008), human modes of gestural communication owe much of their unique complexity to the shared communicative "context." For humans, this context is not simply everything that exists in the immediate environment (temperature, sounds, colours), but everything that is "relevant" for social interaction, i.e. what each participant in the exchange perceives as relevant, knowing that the other perceives it as such. This kind of intersubjective context may be defined as a "joint attentional frame" (Tomasello 2008). Moreover, in all types of human communication, the relationship between overt communicative acts and common terrain, of whatever type, is inversely proportional. That is, the more shared material exists between communicator and recipient, the less need there is to express overt communicative acts (Tomasello 2008, p. 79).

Another point highlighted by Tomasello that is interesting for our argument is linked to the motivation that animates the cooperative spirit with which human beings work to transmit their own messages effectively.

The first and most obvious is "making requests": that is, inducing others to do something useful to us.

The second fundamental human communicative motivation, apparently exclusive to our species, has the purpose of "offering help," sometimes without a request having been made beforehand, providing the other with information that it is thought may be helpful. Applying Searle's (1999) formula to the field of socialisation, Tomasello suggests that "making requests" reflects a "You–I" direction of adaptation, while giving information would reflect an "I–You" direction, since in this case it is the communicator who offers to fit themselves to the needs and desires of the recipient.

Tomasello identifies the third motivation to communicate as a motivation to "share": the communicator wants the recipient to perceive something in a way that makes it possible to share attitudes, but also feelings, so as to increase the common terrain between self and other.

In the sphere of the cognitive neurosciences it has traditionally been maintained that the meaning of a linguistic expression is understood, independently of its context, thanks to the activation of a-modal, symbolic mental representations (Fodor 1998). According to an alternative hypothesis, however, linguistic comprehension would be founded on "embodied" mechanisms, i.e. tied to the body (Lakoff and Johnson 1980; Gallese 2003; Gallese and Lakoff 2005).

According to the "embodied" approach, the same neural structures that govern the organisation of motor execution of actions also play a role in semantic comprehension of the linguistic expressions that describe them. Thanks to embodied simulation, we not only witness an action, emotion, or sensation but, in parallel to this, internal representations of the bodily states associated with these same actions, emotions, and sensations are generated in the observer, "as if" they themselves were performing a similar action or feeling a similar emotion or sensation.

The theory of embodied simulation (Gallese 2003, 2005, 2006; Gallese and Sinigaglia 2011) calls into question the idea that the sole definition of intersubjectivity consists of explicitly attributing propositional attitudes, such as beliefs and desires, to others, mapped as symbolic representations. First, and fundamental to reading other people's minds, there is *intercorporeality* as the principal source of knowledge that we derive directly from others (Gallese 2007; Ammaniti and Gallese 2014).

A number of psychoanalytic authors see the body as a mediator of non-verbal communication, a "representational organ," in the service of the "thing-representation" that is the exclusive perquisite of the unconscious. From this perspective, everything that concerns bodily expression must consequently be imagined as a shortcut by which instincts, affects, and unconscious fantasies speak, bypassing any symbolic system, making themselves present, as it were, to the senses (Di Benedetto 2000). Given that the unconscious emotional message is substantially pre-linguistic, it will not be possible to receive it purely on the verbal level, so it must also reside on the bodily level: as Di Benedetto writes, "an apparently senseless sign receives sense through the senses" (Di Benedetto 2000). Since its foundation, psychoanalysis has universally been considered a talking cure; without speech we could not think of a relationship between a patient and their analyst. Even my son, at the age of 4, when asked what his mother did, replied, "Mamma talks to people."

But if the patient sometimes "lacks" speech, and if the relational space collapses because signification and thought are not possible, the analyst too may lack speech (Racalbuto 1994). So that is where events, acts, and words apparently void of sense can situate themselves: those that seem, and sometimes are, the simple expression of motor discharge, or movements of the body that carry a multiple semantic halo: sometimes these are "enactments" of a traumatic memory which cannot be remembered, at other times thoughts still without a thinker, and at others pre-symbolic traces of a psychic apparatus deprived early on of an *Other* who is capable of signifying. In this collapsed space from which signifying speech is excluded, the "knowing" of verbal representations seems to lose its sense (Racalbuto 1994). There are moments in analysis when the patient as "body" speaks more than the patient as "speech" (Racalbuto 1994, p. 46), obliging the analyst to contain, sometimes for long periods, countertransferential states made of a potent and asymbolic "somatic" affectivity, before they can be transformed into something that may be put into words and shared. They are the cases where an identification with an affect is needed, requiring the analyst to work through in themselves the patient's unrepresentable nucleus that is connected to that affect.

Giulia: A powerful and irresistible drive to represent

In the brief clinical example I will talk about now, the body dominates the scene; one of the specific problems in this patient's treatment consisted in her apparent

inability to gain access to a symbolic-metaphorical function of the mind, understood as a fundamental structure of the unconscious psychological process (Modell
2003, 2009). As a result of this, the patient's unconscious remained trapped in a
body that had no words, and this was a trial for the analytic instrument.

Much of the work prior to a genuine analysis was employed in reactivating a
symbolic-representative function and authentically elaborative thought in the patient. I will only use a brief extract from this long and complex treatment, to illustrate in particular the patient's tendency to *act in the body* as an extreme attempt
to give form to her internal world, while at the same time blocking the way to the
intrusion of the Other by setting up an impenetrable body-mind fortress (Guerrini
Degl'Innocenti 2015).

Giulia was a young adult with anorexic tendencies and a robotic functioning
that entailed an almost total inability to give psychic form to her internal states.
When I met her she had just turned 20 and her body was skeletal: something hard
to look at but at the same time hard to look away from. Her body's ability to attract and hold one's attention went hand in hand with her inability to express any
emotion, to talk about herself. Giulia did not even seem able to turn events into an
autobiographical narrative, and the impossibility of developing a good capacity for
symbolisation was manifest from the start in her complete lack of a language for
representing affects, sensations, and internal states in a full and meaningful manner. In other words, her history, which could not become a story, was dry and empty
of life like her body, coming out of her mouth in disconnected bits as if it had not
been thought about before, as if it had never even been lived. Her primary environment seemed to have been one of those that mix physical and empathic absence,
inconsistency, and failure of mirroring responses, and her primary object appeared
to be unpredictable, intrusive, and unable to tolerate even the idea of separateness.

For a long time I found myself being scrutinised by her as she looked for a response about whatever was currently preoccupying her: sometimes the questions
were implicit, at other times she asked them directly. The distinctive feature of her
questions lay in the fact that what she wanted to know was not my opinion of her,
but "why she was thinking a certain thing" or "what she should do in that situation." Her thoughts did not seem to be representations of reality, but real objects,
facts. There were times when Giulia was terrifying, not just because of the mute
tenacity with which she starved her body (*the body she had*, not *the body she was*),
but also because of the dismaying poverty of her stories, the narrowness of her
relational horizon and, above all, the apparent lack of any emotional sonority or
affective nuance in her language. For a long time the main effort was devoted to
challenging Giulia's continual urge to give up thinking, accommodating most of
the analytic process in my own mind, offering her small bites from barely cooked
dishes made out of basic ingredients which she provided, and whose emotional
content was low.

Proceeding analytically with patients like Giulia, who are extremely concrete in
their thinking and whose language is impoverished, characterised by the inability

to experience a metaphor as a metaphor, requires, sometimes for long periods, a slow patient work of recognising and sharing emotional states as they manifest themselves beyond words. This recognition is achieved by an equally slow but tenacious effort to distinguish the self from the not-self, to reacquaint the body with the affects, helping the patient to build an inner centre endowed with initiative and referentiality. These characteristics of the patient made it necessary to keep any transference interpretation to the minimum because Giulia was incapable of catching the powerfully metaphorical sense of communication in the transference and so my words would have conveyed my thought concretely rather than metaphorically, with the same effect as the way her parents looked at her in a dream from the second year of analysis: something alien and familiar at the same time, which can neither be expelled nor integrated, and can drive you mad.

Towards the end of the third year of therapy, the slow but visible progress of our work together began, on the one hand, to put Giulia back in touch with what was happening in her body, but, on the other, was experienced by her as a danger. Despite the care with which I tried only to cook what she asked me for (for example, avoiding any subject that had not been *introduced* by her), our exchanges, which contained my words and thoughts, nevertheless conveyed the always potentially annihilating and persecutory presence of the other. However, I also think that thanks to these exchanges her mind was beginning to acquire more effective instruments for defence and that this could enable the body slowly to recover some of its vital function, although in compulsive and often dramatic ways. The revitalisation of the body inevitably means instinctual reawakening, libidinal energy in search of recognition and realisation: in other words, a potent and irresistible drive to represent herself to herself which, for Giulia, could at the same time mean intolerable vulnerability to intrusion by the other/the alien.

After an improvement in the clinical picture and the start of some psychic movement, Giulia produced an enigmatic and potent symptom *in the body*: two episodes involving a fall and consequent bruising which, after many uncertainties and an admission to hospital, were diagnosed as epilepsy with no neurological evidence to clarify its origin. I felt divided in two: I was *concretely* worried that this could be something organic and at the same time felt that, *speaking symbolically*, this was not a symptom to be *cured* but the still unformed and tumultuous expression of a need in search of someone *to take care of it*.

After some months of these episodes Giulia started talking in a session about the difficulty she had in knowing what she experienced but, in a different way from usual, she tried with my help to gather up what she seemed to be feeling or knowing about herself, rather as if she were putting together the pieces of a puzzle. We carried on like this for a while, with her putting together and reflecting as I *passed her some pieces* that I had collected for her. Then she stopped and asked:

"Doctor, have you ever had the feeling that your head is empty?"

I replied that there might be more than one reason for this, and that perhaps it could help us to find our way if we knew how she felt, having an empty head.

She answered that it wasn't at all pleasant, and it happened when she decided to think about herself.

I told her that, in my opinion, thinking about herself was unpleasant because it seemed to put her in contact with a sense of emptiness.

She said yes, it had been happening quite often lately, but it was a new thing, maybe like thinking about herself. She was silent for a few minutes and then said:

"I feel like I'm newly born and don't know how to organise my thoughts, as if I don't know how my mind works."

I was struck by what was the first real expression of symbolic/metaphorical thought that Giulia had ever produced in a session, and at the same time I thought about the epileptic seizures. Two different images came into my mind in quick succession: a computer that has to be reset because a virus has invaded it, and a birth where the baby falls to the ground because no one is there to catch it.

I decided as usual to keep these two images in my mind, to make them work for a while with the material that Giulia would bring to subsequent sessions.

In a session a few months later, she told me about very bad headaches that she seemed to suffer from cyclically, and how she'd like to free herself from the pain and from all those thoughts that were taking up all the room and stopping her from functioning.

I told her that perhaps she'd like to treat her head like a computer: to be able to turn it off when it wasn't working properly and switch it back on when it had been reset.

She looked at me in amazement and said yes, that was exactly how she'd like her head to work: *on–off*.

I said to her that maybe those blackouts she had had some months before were her attempt to reset her mind, a way of expelling all that stuff that was taking up room, not allowing her to function, and causing her so much pain.

To conclude

The transformation we are looking for during an analysis is dual: transforming action into language, and transforming the use of language in a way that can support symbolic thought (Birksted-Breen 2012). Psychoanalysis finds itself more and more often dealing with a vast area of manifestations *that do not yet have words* (sensory traces, somatic manifestations, muscular movements, actions) but may, at the same time, have a potent communicative valence. These actions, capable of conveying a meaning and amenable to the attainment of a symbolic function thanks to the potential and transformative space created by the analytic device, are to be understood as *language-actions* whose dramatic freight is aimed at *representing a mental fact* and is located in the *scenic space* (Riolo 1978).

In this particular type of action that I would call *representations in action*, the function of transforming reality intrinsic in the act and from which its communicative function derives, does not disappear – as it does in exclusively expulsive acting – but may encounter the analyst's mind in the transferential–countertransferential scenario. My hypothesis is that these *enactments* are an extreme attempt to give form to the formless in situations where the representational capacity is damaged. This damage, linked to early inadequacies in the function of maternal reverie, prevents the transformation of the emotions that thus invade the psyche in their rawest state, disorganising any possibility of thought. In these cases, the discharge into the outside is not an attempt to expel a harmful or painful thought, but the consequence of the impossibility of producing thought. The *enactment* thus appears to be at the same time a *character in search of an author* and a way to avoid the *psychic constipation* produced by the impossibility of metabolising the raw sensory experience. Moreover, most of the authors who have dealt with the preverbal phases of development and proto-mental configurations emphasise that many of the memories we are concerned with in analysis may, to some extent, be memories "to be constructed" as genuine mental events, repeatedly presenting themselves, enacted, as procedural schemata (Falci 2002), *memories in feelings* (Klein 1957) or *emotional memories* (Weiss 1942). In these cases analytic work specifically means composing the conditions for representability, work that moves through the analyst's engagement, their countertransferential receptiveness, and their capacity for containment and reverie (Barale 1996). In the analytic session, dream-thought understood as a function of the conscious–unconscious mind that is always active in sleep as well as waking (Hautmann 1981; Ferro 2010), can provide the basic thought for the *enactment* that patient and analyst continually nurture, signalling an emergent first level of organisation of the symbolic. This particular modality of thought, which gives rise to dreams in sleep and waking reverie, is the product of an incessant activity by the alpha function which Bion called the *contact barrier* (Bion 1962). This structure-function which creates the conscious and the unconscious, continually separating them and selectively unifying them, enables an incessant proliferation of alpha elements on, we could say, *both sides of the membrane*: on the one hand, it restrains those that remain unconscious and provide the *psychic humus* and, on the other, allows those α-elements necessary for the process of symbolisation to pass into consciousness. If we look from this perspective at the work done with patients like Daniel and Giulia who, in their inability to represent, force the analyst to fulfil the function of symbolic transformation for a long time, we can say that a process has occurred from the starting point of the stimuli coming from the patient, which the analyst's mind has integrated and worked through. Sometimes this process culminated in an interpretative hypothesis which slowly organised itself in my mind and which, from time to time, I decided to translate into a verbal communication to the patient. In step with this, a multitude of ideational, sensory, and emotional stimuli were continually aggregated and redispersed, thereby sustaining, *on the other side of the membrane*, the unconscious figurative potential of the analytic apparatus. During the process, this figurative potential, which the setting and the analytic apparatus made *transitionally* accessible thanks to the establishing of an interpsychic space, generated psychic objects in the form of reveries, metaphors, and dreams. The containing and digestive function of the analyst's mind, which I have tried to illustrate in the clinical material, is the expression of the transference being used for assimilation, metabolisation, and intrapsychic transformation, rather than for unveiling and sharing with the patient, for as long as takes until the symbolic/representative capacities are reactivated and an alphabetisation is possible. In the psychoanalytic exchange with these patients, this *reverberation time* (Birksted-Breen 2005) which, in the mother's psyche, corresponds to the persistence of raw beta elements and their transformation into elements that the baby is able to assimilate, may have a long duration in which the analyst is forced to contain the projections for months or even years before the transformation can happen. Prematurely implementing an interpretation with patients who have experienced obstructive primary objects, communicating a reverie to a patient who has not yet developed sufficient alpha function, or giving a metaphor to a patient who is not capable of producing their own, may carry the risk of transforming an *inter-psychic exchange* into a *trans-psychic intrusion* (Bolognini 2010) and once more occluding the natural human *drive to represent*.

Note

1 The reference is to the 1983 film and its post-nuclear holocaust scenario.

References

Ambrosiano L. (2009). Con la realtà addosso. *Rivista di Psicoanalisi* 55, 303–324.
Ammaniti M. and Gallese V. (2014). La nascita della intersoggettività. Lo sviluppo del Sé tra psicodinamica e neurobiologia. Raffaello Cortina Editore, Milan.
Barale F. (1996). "Si prega di chiudere gli/un occhi(o)": appunti su agire e ricordare. *Rivista di Psicoanalisi* 42, 425–453.
Birksted-Breen D. (2005). Il tempo e l'après-coup. *L'Annata Psicoanalitica Internazionale* 1, 13–28.
Birksted-Breen D. (2012). Taking Time: The Tempo of Psychoanalysis. *International Journal of Psychoanalysis* 93, 819–835.
Blatt S.J. (1974). Levels of Object Representation in Anaclitic and Introjective Depression. *Psychoanalytic Study of the Child* 29, 107–157.
Bion W. (1962). *Learning from Experience*. Karnac, London, 1984.
Bion W.R. (1973). *Brazilian Lectures*. Karnac, London, 1990.
Bollas C. (1995). *Cracking Up: the Work of Unconscious Experience*. Routledge, London.
Bolognini S. (2008). *Secret Passages: The Theory and Technique of Interpsychic Relations*. Routledge, Hove, 2011.
Bolognini S. (2010). Passaggi segreti verso l'inconscio: stili e tecniche di interpretazione. *Rivista di Psicoanalisi* 56, 599–613.
Botella C. and Botella S. (2001). *The Work of Psychic Figurability: Mental States Without Representation*. Brunner-Routledge, Hove, 2005.
Campbell D. and Enckell H. (2005). Metaphor and the violent act. *International Journal of Psychoanalysis* 86, 801–823.
Di Benedetto A. (2000). *Prima della parola. L'ascolto psicoanalitico del non detto attraverso le forme dell'arte*. Franco Angeli Editore, Rome.
Falci A. (2002). La competenza comunicativa e la sua influenza nella terapia analitica.

Rivista di Psicoanalisi 48, 873–887.

Ferro A. (2010). *Torments of the Soul: Psychoanalytic Transformations in Dreaming and Narration*. Routledge, Hove, 2015

Ferruta A. (2013). Setting analitico e spazio per l'altro. *Rivista di Psicoanalisi* 59, 607–622.

Filippini S. and Zavattini G.C. (1999). *Il mondo rappresentazionale: Joseph Sandler*. In Lis A., Stella S. and Zavattini G.C. (eds.) *Manuale di psicologia dinamica*. Il Mulino, Bologna.

Fodor J.A. (1998). *Concepts: Where Cognitive Science Went Wrong*. Oxford University Press, Oxford.

Freud S. (1887–1904). *The Complete Letters of Sigmund Freud to Wilhelm Fliess*. Masson J. M. (ed.). Harvard, Cambridge MA, 1986.

Freud S. (1895). Project for a Scientific Psychology. SE, 1.

Freud S. (1899). *The Interpretation of Dreams*. SE, 4–5.

Freud S. (1911). Formulations on the Two Principles of Mental Functioning. SE, 12.

Freud S. (1914). Remembering, Repeating and Working-Through. SE, 12.

Freud S. (1923). *The Ego and the Id*. SE, 19.

Freud S. (1925). Negation. SE, 19.

Gaddini E. (1984). Se e come sono cambiati i nostri pazienti fino ai nostri giorni. *Rivista di Psicoanalisi* 30, 560–580.

Gallese V. (2003). The Roots of Empathy: The Shared Manifold Hypothesis and the Neural Basis of Intersubjectivity. *Psychopathology* 36, 171–180.

Gallese V. (2005). *Being Like Me: Self-Other Identity, Mirror Neurons and Empathy*. In Harley S. and Chater N. (ed) *Perspectives on Imitation: From Cognitive Neuroscience to Social Science*, vol. 1. MIT Press, Cambridge MA, 101–118.

Gallese V. (2006). Intentional Attunement: A Neurophysiological Perspective on Social Cognition and its Disruption in Autism. *Brain Research* 1079, 15–24.

Gallese V. (2007). Before and Below Theory of Mind: Embodied Simulation and the Neural Correlates of Social Cognition. *Philosophical Transactions of the Royal Society B: Biological Sciences* 362, 659–669.

Gallese V. and Lakoff G. (2005). The Brain Concepts: The Role of the Sensory-Motor System in Conceptual Knowledge. *Cognitive Neuropsychology* 21, 1–25.

Gallese V. and Sinigaglia C. (2011). What is so Special with Embodied Simulation? *Trends in Cognitive Sciences* 15, 512–519.

Giaconia G., Pellizzari G. and Rossi P. (2008). *Identità ed entropia del soggetto*. XIV Congresso SPI Giornate Italiane, Rome, 22–25 May 2008.

Gilbert C. (1989). *On Social Facts*. International Library of Philosophy Series, Princeton University Press, Princeton.

Green A. (1975). *Psicoanalisi degli stati limite. La follia privata*. Cortina Editore, Milan, 1991.

Green A. (2002). *Key Ideas for a Contemporary Psychoanalysis*. London, Routledge, 2005.

Guerrini Degl'innocenti B. (2015). L'inconscio incarnato. Sull'uso della rêverie e della metafora nel trattamento di una paziente anoressica. *Rivista di Psicoanalisi* 61, 293–313.

Hautmann G. (1981). Il mio debito con Bion: dalla psicoanalisi come teoria alla psicoanalisi come funzione della mente. *Rivista di Psicoanalisi* 27, 558–572.

Klein M. (1957). *Envy and Gratitude and Other Works*. London, Hogarth, 1975.

Lakoff G. and Johnson M. (1980). *Metaphors We Live By*. Chicago University Press.

Modell A.H. (2003). *Imagination and the Meaningful Brain*. Bradford Books, MIT Press, Cambridge, MA.

Modell A.H. (2009). Metaphor – The Bridge Between Feelings and Knowledge. *Psychoanalytic Inquiry* 29, 6–11.

Piaget J. and Inhelder B. (1966). *The Psychology of the Child*. Basic Books, New York 1969.

Quinodoz D. (2005). Parole che toccano. *L'Annata Psicoanalitica Internazionale* 1, 165–181.

Racalbuto A. (1994). Tra il fare e il dire. Raffaello Cortina Editore, Milan.

Riolo F. (1978). L'"agire" come linguaggio e rappresentazione. *Rivista di Psicoanalisi* 24, 364–378.

Roussillon R. (2015). Un'introduzione al lavoro sulla simbolizzazione primaria. *Rivista di Psicoanalisi* 2, 479–491.

Ruggiero I. (2017). *Quale posto per l'azione nella relazione analitica?* In Ruggiero I. and Rossi N. (eds.) *La relazione psicoanalitica. Contributi clinici e teorici*. Franco Angeli Editore, Rome.

Sandler, J. (1990). On Internal Object Relations. *Journal of the American Psychoanalytic Association* 38, 859–879.

Sandler J. and Rosenblatt B. (1962). *Il concetto di mondo rappresentazionale*. In Sandler J. *La ricerca in psicoanalisi*, Vol. 1. Boringhieri, Turin, 1980.

Scarfone D. (2013). From Faces to Signs. In Levine H.B., Reed G.S. and Scarfone D. (eds.) *Unrepresented States and the Construction of Meaning*. Karnac, London.

Schafer R. (1968). *Aspects of Internalization*. International Universities Press, New York.

Searle J.R. (1999). *Mind, Language and Society*. Basic Books, New York, 2008.

Tomasello M. (2008). *Origins of Human Communication*. MIT: Cambridge, MA.

Tomasello M., Carpenter M., Call J., Behne T. and Moll H. (2005). Understanding and sharing intentions: The origins of cultural cognition. *Behavioral and Brain Sciences* 28, 675–735.

Weiss E. (1942). Emotional Memories and Acting Out. *Psychoanalytic Quarterly* 11, 477–492.

Winnicott D.W. (1965). *Maturational Processes and the Facilitating Environment: Studies in the Theory of Emotional Development*. Hogarth, London.

Wittgenstein L. (1953). *Philosophical Investigations*. Wiley-Blackwell, Chichester, 2009.

Chapter 3

Openings for listening to words

Anna Ferruta

Overture – a clearing in the forest of symbols

We can use the psychoanalytic method to "test" some critical manifestations of psychic life that seem to elude it and make their actualisation arduous or impossible. Sometimes a profound suffering compels the patient to ask the analyst an urgent, pressing question that admits no delay because of the intensity of long-denied, dissociated, imprisoned emotions. These are preverbal experiences, lived but not symbolised and integrated, which are on the point of bursting out, destroying psychic functioning and causing fractures in relations with the familial and social environment (self-harm/harm to others, or requests for immediate sedation to restore the previous silent state and eliminate the anxiety which is felt as being brought by a foreign guest who has just turned up). They are primary affective experiences that often communicate by means other than language and have been left unintegrated within the overall functioning of the personality, which has evaded them by performing a kind of slalom. It sometimes happens that these processes of avoidance are no longer possible, for example at the arrival of the adolescent period, when the desire for physical and emotional contact with the other-than-self is urgently manifest, or when traumatic situations compel the subject to pass through the door that had been avoided by the skilful slalom of life (bereavements, retirement, changes of location, abandonments, etc.).

Youthful breakdown and the dissociative crises of middle age often indicate reactions to an impoverishment of the Self and the relationships, hidden until that moment under the narcissistic set-up of material wellbeing or adequate forms of behaviour. From this viewpoint, there is a particularly significant difference between an approach directed towards resolving the symptomatic and behavioural emergency, and analytic listening in the analysing situation (Roussillon 2018) aimed at accommodating and giving a voice to the other in the self and in the object.

Analytic listening is open to detecting the deficiency in the processes of subjectivating primary experiences based on affect and not yet on articulate language, and to offering a psychic space for going to meet what one does not yet know, by means of listening to that "dissemination" that Bollas (1995) talks about, which is the opposite of the processes of avoidance and phobia. This "emergence" of

DOI: 10.4324/9781003544647-3

unconscious contents via the weakening of defensive set-ups can be welcomed by an analytic mind instead of being diverted elsewhere, towards pharmacological or supportive provisions aimed at instantly switching off the demand for help that has made itself felt through symptoms, anxieties, acts. It is a matter of developing the conditions for listening analytically to these emerging phenomena, containing the over-eagerness to integrate them straightaway in the personality as a whole.

In psychoanalysis we need to keep the appropriate conditions constant so that unconscious communications can take place and transformations can unite cognitions, affects, and senses. This is one of the problems with widening the boundaries of contemporary psychoanalysis: the abstract formula "anything goes" is no more valid than the repetition of rigid canons.

We are asking how to widen the capacity for treatment and for psychoanalytic knowledge without it becoming a disembodied meta-philosophy or an adaptive therapeutic practice, but instead maintaining its quality as a method that helps to expand subjectivity, generative encounters with the other-than-oneself, and acquaintance with what is unknown about oneself and the other. This is an arduous task, to which an alert clinical practice and open-minded theoretical reflection are trying to make a contribution, digging into the heart of psychoanalysis and the sufferings of our contemporary world.

Equipment that helps to encounter reality and hitherto inaccessible psychic ways of functioning is a fundamental aspect of psychoanalytic experiences. Our therapeutic knowledge and capacities are also extended thanks to the use of instruments such as the transference, countertransference, reverie, free associations, and listening without memory and desire in the therapeutic context with non-neurotic patients encountered in pre-arranged settings that allow the analysing situation to be activated.

Some deeper investigations into the quality of analytic listening act as fundamental points of reference which have widened our capacity for contact with the unconscious dimensions of psychic life. These are our starting points: for example, the Winnicott (1966) of "I am listening to a girl," when he notices the mental position he finds himself in unconsciously while thinking that his patient (a man) is talking to him about penis envy. Winnicott emphasises the importance of listening attentively to dissociated parts that make themselves perceptible to listening in the analytic situation. Another necessary starting point is Bion (1967), who invites the analyst to listen "without memory or desire" because the only important thing in any session is what is not known, and it is essential to let this emerge from the darkness and evolve on the basis of the relational experience between two single subjects. We also need to start from Haydée Faimberg's (1981) "listening to listening," which invites the analyst to catch the way the patient has listened or not listened to the analyst's communication, as an essential element of the interaction between unconsciouses that unfolds in the analytic session. And we need to start from the "respectful listening" of Luciana Nissim Momigliano (1992) who thinks that, in the training of psychoanalytic pupils, it is important for the analyst to be decentred and learn the dialect spoken by the patient.[1]

Based on these fundamental conceptual openings, we go on *looking for new instruments that may enable us to know aspects of psychic functioning* unknown until now: as indeed happens in fields of science, from endoscopy to PET, to MRI, etc. By its nature, psychoanalysis involves refining the instrument of the encounter between two subjects in the field of their unconscious communications, creating a space-time for a subjective experience in contact with another person.

The psychoanalytic experience is experience of the unconscious and its effects on subjectivity within an apparatus that makes those effects emerge to be encountered, captured, and interpreted.

So we need to link and systematise the devices that make unconscious psychic reality emerge. In particular, this complex nexus (instruments, settings, pathologies) has enabled us to enlarge the conception of the unconscious, which includes not only processes connected to the traces of bodily experience and of significant relationships, but also unconscious processes lacking organisation, whose contents also depend on the contingent interpersonal field which activates them and gives them form and existence, often in a dramatic and theatrical way. The activation of unconscious processes also depends profoundly on the availability of another subject to animate them, in every sense.

The analytic relationship offered in a profoundly interpersonal dimension that puts the emotions and associations of patient and analyst in play, superseding the attention oriented selectively towards the dynamic aimed at reconstructing childhood experiences, acts as a field in which events occur and come into being, events that enable the development of experiential potentialities not yet utilised. After long periods of routine and stagnation, silences and repetitions, suddenly moments of meeting are sparked, linked to the analyst's timing and readiness to listen. Such moments create a transformative context that does not follow logically from what has happened previously, but encounters a caesura, an indescribable movement between diachrony and synchrony in the analytic process.

This opening of horizons depends on the prearranging of conditions favourable to the development of knowledges that are fully immersed in clinical experience: the indispensable generative matrix is the nexus between advances in theory (widening the space of meanings), settings that make it possible to activate the analysing situation, and an encounter with primal psychic experiences. This can happen in situations that are open to "emergings," both in a first meeting and over the course of a long analysis, as if a clearing had opened during a dark journey in the forest, as was represented by a patient's dream in a similar context.

Absolute listening "not greedy" for meanings

The process of becoming a subject unfolds in relation to an otherness that is to be encountered, and from the outset offers an absolute welcome, open to listening to moments of subjectivity which still have neither subject nor object, listening to that which is neither thing nor word but nevertheless communication of the self. In the analytic situation a listening is activated, made of a suspended attention on the part of the analyst, ready to be astonished, to fail to understand, and not to throw itself avidly into the clutches of a meaning that could be possessed for narcissistic gratification. An "absolute" listening, freed from ties to meanings, open to any form of signifier and made of passion for otherness in its nascent state: a listening that may be welcoming but not immediately imprisoned in a relationship where the object would end up occupying most of the space with its claim to be wise and indispensable.

Enzo Morpurgo (1988, 1998) is one of the psychoanalysts who have gone deepest in talking about analytic listening by therapists who are capable of welcoming the patient's suffering instead of denying it:

> It seems that such people, sometimes bonded by a peer relationship, are free of "tension," endowed with a welcoming inner space but not of the kind that "takes hold forever," and are equipped with a silent openness to the outside world, potentially active, but not greedy. They are people endowed with a "lengthening" of the mental capacity for sounding the minds of others without wounding or dominating them.
>
> (Morpurgo 1998, p. 78)

Morpurgo thinks that this readiness to listen, a listening as "absolute" as the musical ear, embodies a "matrix of the therapeutic position." This absolute listening, free from pre-constituted, pre-categorial nexuses, is aimed at detecting the subject where it has not been able to constitute itself as different from the habitual Self imprisoned in the tangle of defences and splits. Every individual is a plurality of transmitters, often in conflict with each other, waiting for a listener who can detect them and make them audible to the individual as well.

The function of the other as an attentive listener is fundamental: of course, it is true that emotions which have been obstructed in their emergence to the surface of consciousness acquire life and form in the unconscious dimension as dreams, but dreams predominantly activate the visual functions which rely on a certain "social" consensuality with the other-than-self, even when the images are drawn from abstract or informal art, or *arte povera*. When the analyst's listening is turned predominantly toward sonic communication, it situates itself in a dimension less structured by a validating anticipatory consensuality and aims to catch moments of subjectivity without a subject that emerge by using the vehicle of the word and at the same time indicate an inner condition of desire to develop a relationship with an other-than-self.

Jean-Luc Donnet believes that the almost fetishistic aura with which analytic listening is charged "is linked to the counter-suggestive requirement of the method *per via di levare* invented by Freud: if listening is only receptive, if it just makes an echo, it does not risk 'suggesting,' operating *per via di porre*" (Donnet 2008, § 1).[2] The analyst pays the same evenly suspended attention to everything the patient offers, whereas an intentional attention would inevitably be selective.

The wager of the fundamental rule is that by doing away with any object defined or agreed beforehand it ensures that the session is left with the task of simultaneously ensuring both the production and the investigation of "the unconscious object." This object is thus first of all the very process of the session ... It is the listening which, making a choice at a given moment, retroactively constitutes the object of interpretation.

(Donnet 2008, § 5)

Michael Parsons underlines the special and specific quality of this listening by the analyst, who is not greedy to appropriate meanings:

Interpretations which abstract a patient's meaning run the same risk as academic commentaries on poetry: the risk of appropriating meaning to themselves while the breath of life in the original is lost. Because reality in the internal analytic setting is defined by unconscious meaning, it is within the internal setting that an analyst can best simply hear meaning without needing to abstract it.

(Parsons 2007, p. 1445)

The sonic material of island-words

I want to go further in search of the elements that compose this analytic listening, first of all highlighting the sense of hearing as a whole: the patient's communication is sonic material, a vibration of the air that reaches the eardrum, which vibrates in turn and transmits messages via the acoustic nerves. Freud had already asserted this, with a great proleptic intuition of future developments: "In essence a word is after all the mnemic residue of a word that has been heard" (Freud 1923, p. 21). Sound is a concrete fact that reaches the analyst independently of meaning: it is the noise of the intentional desire to communicate, which in the presence of the analyst begins to function and to become the expressive vehicle of a subjectivity *in fieri*. It is sonic material that the analyst is willing to welcome *a priori* with joy, before even knowing its content, as in the finale of the film by Richard Brooks, *Deadline* (1952): when the crime boss asks, "What's that noise?" the journalist played by Humphrey Bogart answers, "That's the press, baby, the press." It is the noise of the machines printing the newspaper that he is finally able to "publish," making himself heard after resisting the threats of mafiosi who wanted to shut him down and silence him.

In psychoanalysis the auditory dimension is privileged over the visual, for more than one reason: while it is communication between unconsciouses that is waiting to be activated and made accessible, we know that the visual dimension is more structured and responds immediately to Gestalt parameters which organise the perceived scene according to exploratory schemata that are helpful but still partly "bound" by the history of the previous perceptions that have been effective in orienting us in the world.[3] By contrast, listening to sonic material occurs via a sensory dimension like the auditory, less structured and more disposed to be perceived as not-known, not understood, and not organised into representational schemata predefined by colour, form, content. The analyst is willing to listen to sonic communications which begin by signalling the presence of a subject *in fieri* that desires to be grasped, without a prejudicial foreclosure of their sufficiency and meaning.

To become a subject and achieve a subjective appropriation of the world we need encounters with alterities that make space for a sometimes silent subject *in fieri*, sometimes in a state of flat calm while waiting for the encounter with a "thinking heart" (Alvarez 2012), and at other times overflowing with an excess of sensoriality which in its exuberance obstructs the communicative emergence towards an Other who may be able to understand it. What is necessary is the willing aptitude for sonic listening, even listening to the sound of silence – which is never not sound – without setting off a lust for plunder and without the uncontainable eagerness to fill disorienting pauses and gaps. As Morpurgo (1998) writes, the analyst can begin by catching the patient's desire to be perceived, this generative readiness to be felt as existing, despite everything.

Poet and psychoanalyst Adriana Pagnoni uses her poetry to describe this desire to be listened to as a tragic dimension of "being-not" (*Essere non. Il bilico dell'esistenza* [Being-not. Existence as balance.]), the desire for a listening that does not seal off the essential void of the "not" of being which runs away as soon as it has been detected as "being-not," wishing it hadn't let itself be perceived in the communication, despite everything. This risk-desire of someone to be detected in the analytic communication is indicated by Adriana Pagnoni (2000) in several poems as the sudden appearance of a red light that bursts out like a word endowed with a particular intensity, like a warning light about the danger of being imprisoned in the representational world of the other, the analyst, and thus annulled and defeated in the Sisyphean labour of becoming a subject, the struggle to appropriate something of the other that might contribute to the individual's feeling existent in relation to their own and the other's otherness:

"*I am / the letter / not received / the bread I lacked / in childhood / my father's / non-return / the little red / bike I dreamed.*"

Adriana Pagnoni has succeeded in expressing in the most succinct way, in the fewest possible words made of essential sounds and ordinary content, like the colour word "red," a sense of profound inner revolt against an archaic unconscious imposition not to live a subjectivated existence, to be a "being-not." But from this imprisoning constriction, kept at bay with the clenched teeth of silence, island-words continually escape, filling the page with objects from life that run away and present themselves again with the authority of the senses: a little red bicycle to escape on, a ball caught but then allowed to roll away:

"*Bloody / red / of red / blood / the hand that / on waking / still / holds / the red / in flight / of the ball / caught / in the dream.*"

In "absolute" analytic listening the analyst is reached and struck by these isolated *island-words* that emerge in a communication which follows a logic other than that of speech and are looking for another person to catch and hold them, someone who won't let them be dispersed into the clouds like an apparently worthless little red ball, which in fact marks a first possibility of subjectivation, open over the abyss of the analyst's unconscious as she listens to what is "other" than the already known and shared.

Openness to analytic listening is signalled by these island-words which reach the analyst with their sonic and sensory intensity as the sign of an other's presence: "red" is an adjective that has a sonic intensity as well as a plurality of possible associative connections, precisely because of its basic, essential, bloody quality.

This is why, in analytic listening, the sonic material that words are made of, beside their meaning, constitutes the essential element of an acknowledgement of otherness by the analyst, who does not prematurely appropriate the patient's subjective creations to herself, nor cover or fill them with her own imaginative contents, but remains in a musical dimension of listening, in a mutual encounter with an otherness that is to be acknowledged and not wiped out under a mountain of words. Sometimes the classical taut and participatory silence represents an essential component of analytic listening.

The forms of presence of the object that listens

Unconscious communications are activated by the presence of the object, which arouses psychic intensities in a different way from the traces left in the subjective reworking of oneiric activity in dream.

The physical presence of the analyst-object activates and deactivates, animates and destroys the patient's subjectivity. Roussillon (2015) has made an in-depth study of the difference between the presence of the analyst as object–subject and a relationship with the analyst-object. For people with narcissistic-identity problems in particular, the very presence of the other can interfere with the expression and growth of the self. Roussillon has explored the role played by the forms of the object's presence in allowing or obstructing the process of subjectivation. He has developed a detailed theory based on what had earlier been brought to light by Luciana Nissim Momigliano in *L'ascolto rispettoso* [Respectful Listening] (2001) and Haydée Faimberg in *The Telescoping of Generations* (2006).

Luciana Nissim Momigliano (1992) thinks that the analyst should be decentred and make way for the history and world of the patient:

> The people who come to analysis have taught me that for many of them this is the first and last opportunity in their lives to be able to find someone who will finally try to see things as they see them, and to listen to their story: that is, the theory they have made about their life and sufferings, without immediately proposing or imposing their own way of thinking, without judging, devaluing, or mocking them … in short, someone who will feel a sincere interest and a benign curiosity in what they are or think themselves to be.
>
> (Nissim Momigliano 1992, p. 75)

Haydée Faimberg makes an extended analysis of how the patient responds to the analyst's interventions, attuning herself by listening to how the patient has responded, whether as an open pathway to free associations, storytelling, and interaction or as a critic, a limit, a request to intervene no further in the dialogue:

> The analyst focuses his attention on the fate of his interpretation or on the fate of his silence in the patient's psyche. This is what I understand by "the presence of the analyst": to listen and to interpret the destiny of what the patient has heard.
>
> (Faimberg 1981, p. 30)

The presence of the analyst as object–subject, with her physicality and imposing occupation of a place in the patient's room-mind, can be perceived as threatening when, as soon as a faint sign of life has been detected in the patient, the analyst hurls herself on top of it and devours it with her expansive cannibal subjectivity, making it her own with an appreciation and agreement which absorb it into her seraglio. Or else the presence of the analyst-object may be implicitly perceived by the patient as an order to disappear, an injunction to absent himself as a free, active, individual subject, and turn into pure available presence, like a sentry on guard at the royal palace. And so no room is allowed in the analytic space for another subject, but only for an agent whose psychic space is completely occupied by the other in Superegoic military uniform. The mere presence of another person in the same room is an implicit order to disappear, to make way for an object who has the legitimate right to priority. This dynamic can be well described in terms of breathing difficulties caused by the presence of someone else in the same space, which risks a lack of oxygen, induces isolation or prompts a search for infinite spaces of solitude "so one can breathe" (the sea, a desert, a high mountain).

The presence of the other with the word, which reaches the subject as a concrete sonic message, is essential for activating the dimension of unconscious communication and a psychic intensity that may develop the interaction between unconsciouses: but sometimes it is that very presence which obstructs. I recall a subject who periodically needs trips to wide open places with an unobstructed horizon (for example, the open sea in a sailing boat or long hikes in the mountains away from any paths) because the mere encounter with another person brings into the present an implicit task involving something that demands a solution, something ubiquitous that is always potentially present in human affairs (it's hot, it's cold, something has fallen onto the floor, a noise acts as a reminder of the other, etc.).

The object's mode of response in the early phases of life can contribute to the creation of blockages in primary symbolisation which have left space for a relationship based predominantly on *training*, in which subjectivation has not happened. These situations prompt questions about the modes of listening in analysis. Listening that aims to identify and communicate reconstructions of these early failed interactions cannot reach the patient because these "histories" come to him in the pre-emptive and injunctive mode of the experiential context in which he first lived them. On the other hand, silence leaves the patient with an absence of personal elements to be subjectivated because relational intensities are missing. Psychoactive substances are often resorted to so that the situation can be blocked, causing further isolation from the object.

Roussillon (2015) highlights the importance in analysis of capturing early forms of symbolisation like the pictograms of Piera Aulagnier (1975) and the formal signifiers of Didier Anzieu (1994). That is, he believes it is important to extract a formal signifier from the associative chain brought by the patient: to put it another way, we must develop a capacity for listening to the isolated "word" which emerges at the surface of consciousness activated by the interaction with the other, sometimes for its sound alone, at other times because it is out of context, like a messenger from the unconscious that has escaped the prison of the discourse and regained its enigmatic function as Hermes, messenger of the gods.

The analyst's listening can thus be directed to the word as an element that is extraneous to the logical, historical, and signifying landscape of the discourse, as an event that establishes a possibility of subjectivating the patient's unconscious world in a language that sounds strange, out of tune, foreign to the usual communication with the analyst. Different languages are always spoken in analysis, that of the analyst and that of the patient, or rather, the languages of the various characters who emerge in the context of the analytic session, which acts as a theatre, a stage open to the entry of unknown actors into the scene.

Again, Donnet notes the paradoxical condition of analytic listening:

> Listening thus finds itself plugged into the formal regression of thinking and the hallucinatory potential of word-representations on the model of dream-work. In the projective register of the transference enacted in words, listening is gripped by the quasi-hallucinatory quality that regression confers on the highly charged affect.
>
> (Donnet 2008, § 9)

The very business of free association requires patients to detach themselves from the known elements that gave them security and to expose themselves to an encounter with the not-known that may appear in the formal signifier of a disconnected word divorced from the logic of the discourse. Some words become bearers of subjectivations that are still in the process of being completed. Nowadays, in current communication on the various media, the world "hybrid" has made its appearance with an unprecedented frequency (cars, credit cards), which suggests the contradictions that coexist in the mind, possibilities of presence without whole or completed integrations, hybrid psychosomatic dimensions like breath, a vegetative function but one that can also be controlled by consciousness, a function especially afflicted today with impasses between unconscious and conscious, as happens during panic attacks.

Roussillon (2018) indicates how "polyphonic polymorphous heteromorphous listening" employs associative modes which only reveal *the patient's communicative potential once the object has made its response.* These forms of primitive communication do not only consist in states of evacuation or motor expression, but are also attempts to get across to the object the message about the experience of the enigmatic internal state which needs to be integrated.

Intensities of the word

The unconscious manifests itself if it is activated by a presence that arouses psychic intensities. Anne Alvarez (2012) thinks that with certain patients the analyst must be careful not to extinguish their embryonic emotional vitality: sometimes it may be better to avoid indicating who is having the experience and to use impersonal forms of expression when alluding to what is occurring and taking shape. To say, for example, "it is upsetting when …" may be a way to name and describe the experience that is coming to light before clarifying whether there is a subject who can take responsibility for it and acknowledge it as its own, as something being shared with another mind.

Bollas (1992) says that the individual is evoked by encounters with objects which give him or her the opportunity to express and get to know unknown unconscious aspects of the self: we are initiators of our experience and also initiated by our experience, *by desire and by chance.* The existence of an unconscious psychic life that is played out in the encounter with others constitutes a patrimony of inestimable value:

> However well analyzed we may be, we shall always be a subject who only ever partly knows. Partly knows the other. Partly knows the self. Partly knows life. Most of our life is lived unconsciously, in dialogue with the other's unconscious, within the field of unconscious social processes.
>
> (Bollas 1992, pp. 116–117)

The therapist is asked to contain the maximum possible diversity, giving it form, utilising the unknown unconscious space. In doing this, the first meeting with the patient is especially important: the risk for the patient is that this *chance* will be missed, that they will see the opportunity to express potential unconscious aspects, the *desire*, slip through their fingers; and the risk for the therapist is that of reproducing the traumatic familial and environmental conditions when faced with the first manifestations of suffering. As Freud teaches, this is also already an attempt to find a way out of an emotional situation that has become unliveable because it is no longer manageable by repression or other defences (splitting, dissociation, avoidance, denial, isolation). The emotion emerges via the suffering that prompts the hand to reach out in the transference of the first meeting.

Winnicott (1965) believes that when patients have regressed to a state of helpless dependency, as may happen in a first meeting on the brink of a breakdown, any word the therapist may actually say is perceived as seductive and thus as incorporating the subject in the seductive object, or else as persecutory, as an aggressive and intrusive invasion. For the therapist it is a matter of navigating these difficult waters, giving the greatest possible space to listening and to acknowledging the embryonic otherness of the subject who is coming towards her.

An example: I am thinking of Jacob, a young man passionate about astronomy and blocked by the claustrophobic fear of enclosed spaces, beginning with the metro that he needs if he wants to spend time outside the college where he is living while he pursues his study of interstellar spaces as an engineer. At our first meeting this is the communication that I feel is important: "My mother's therapist sent me." His mother is depressed and lives in another city.

In the first meeting it is fundamental to be ready and willing to listen and to catch the living transferential element, the hidden hand held out, the psychic intensity put into play in the relational field: "My mother's therapist sent me." In this communication of Jacob's the diagnosis and the therapy come together, cryptically entwined, a bundle to be caught in flight, and so I need time and commitment to read, understand, and interpret it. It is as if Jacob were saying,

> I can't go out and look for my life, my path, my girlfriend, all these things that I want but are lightyears away, unreachable; I'm the prisoner of a bond I don't want to/can't give up, the desire for a gaze that will notice my existence. Only someone who'll cure my (internal/external) mother and help her to look at me will be able to free me from this imprisonment. For now, I'm like the prisoner who looks at the stars through the bars in the window of his cell.

Naturally all this imagined development of Jacob's news bulletin is the fruit of the work done for a long time together, brought to a conclusion after many years. The important thing in the first meeting was to catch the intensity of the hand held out, the request for both a home and the stars, for closure and flight. A young man from another city, alone and shut away in college, is able to communicate the psychic intensity of his desire to escape imprisonment in a relationship that annuls his existence. So, in the first meeting my mind has various diagnostic configurations fluctuating in it, along with possible forced and premature interpretations. I think I could say to him,

> Perhaps it isn't you who want to start a course of psychotherapy and you feel sent by someone else, who actually isn't interested in you but in your mother: maybe like your father, who is willing to pay for your therapy.

Instead I reject all this: I would become the mother concentrating on my own pre-occupations in the form of an attention oriented towards my prejudicial diagnostic or interpretative categories. So I try to catch hold of the transferential intensity in the communication and say, "It must have been difficult to get this far. We will be able to move together towards new experiences." I only realise afterwards that my first communication happens in an impersonal form ("it must have been difficult"), that it has attended to the communicative intensity being put into play but does not yet configure Jacob as an Ego-subject, who for now is absent.

Condensation of the word

As happens in dream, the dialogue that unfolds between analyst and patient occurs in a pre-arranged space-time, with the deactivation of voluntary motor activity and all assigned tasks. In an analytic session, new rules are activated for the unconscious functioning of communication in the pre-arranged setting, both in its external dimension (regularity of the meetings, suspension of the events of everyday life) and in its internal dimension (activation in the analyst's mind of the dialogue "for the other") "in order to recognise [the other] where they are not, and not recognise them where they have been arrogantly attested in their full deceptiveness" (Morpurgo 1988, p. 198). Communication in free associations and free-floating attention unconsciously follow a grammar and syntax that are somewhat different from those of everyday speech, which is directed towards a declared purpose (e.g. asking a passerby the way: it has a practical purpose, that of achieving a goal, but in the meta-dimension of the analytic setting it would act as a communication of an entirely different kind). Like the dream-work described by Freud in Chapter 6 of *The Interpretation of Dreams* (1900) it follows certain rules that translate dream-thoughts into communicable derivatives (condensation, displacement, symbolic representation, secondary elaboration), so in the analytic session the dialogue follows a course that is not limited to the manifest content, a motion that words burst into with a communicative charge which exceeds the logic of the discourse. They are words whose production follows a principle of condensation similar to the images of a dream: words that come to the surface of consciousness, breaking through the linear atmosphere that is being condensed and introducing affects, emotions, contents, condensations in an intensity of possible associative nexuses that have not yet been fully revealed but have overcome a kind of gravitational force which was keeping them anchored to the depths of the unconscious dimension.

Listening to these "condensed" words is particularly significant because we can detect in them the transformative potential which surfaces in the dialogue, for the sole reason that they have appeared and acquired citizenship in the shared communication. Then, when they re-emerge session by session, they accumulate contents and discourses around themselves, which are to be encountered and dealt with in secondary elaboration. But the most important psychic work happens with their appearance.

From this perspective, particular interest is afforded by the patient's unique personal language which uses words from the analytic interaction as condensations of cognitions and affects, as the dream-elements that become a basis for creating a personal psychic world of his or her own. These words mark the transitions in the analytic work not so much by their semantic significance but because they represent the fruit of an interaction between unconsciouses around which specific elements are consolidated, having flowed out of the spiralling dialogue between fully engaged subjects. In *Free Associations: Memories of a Psychoanalyst*, Ernest Jones tells how "it was Trotter who first mentioned ... a man in Vienna who actually listened with attention to every word his patients said to him" (Jones 1959, p. 149).

The word can be considered in its cognitive, semantic, evocative, and sonic valence or as a complex amalgam of meanings and affects that take on a temporary identitary valence, which is partly out of context and, thanks to the fortunate opportunity of the analysing situation, is able to float to the surface of consciousness and become a distillation of the interpretative and transformative journey.

In a paper about listening and the five senses, Nancy Chodorow (2012) highlights the natural and plural complexity of the word, besides its cognitive value:

> Several colleagues, focused on rhythm and tone as well as on meaning, conceptualize free association as a melding of the words and sounds of poetry into music. Ogden (1999) writes of "'the music of what happens' in poetry and psychoanalysis" Seiden (2004), in "On the Music of Thought," about metaphor in poetry and psychoanalysis, and Jones (1997) of the missing "orchestration" (p. 694) of words, tone, timbre, and emphasis in many case reports.
>
> (Chodorow 2012, p. 754)

We can pay attention to the words used by the patient as elements with which to construct their personal psychic world. They are words that can be used as "compasses" for making progress in the analytic work: I recall a word that began to make its appearance in the speech of a woman who had previously encountered numerous failures in the analytic treatments she had undertaken, being the prisoner of now repetitive mental schemata. Little by little in her speech during sessions the word "pounding" starts to feature with its persecutory charge, but also with its quality of "woody" sonic concreteness which resonates and makes itself noisily felt in the tangle of impasses caused by her intellectualised communication. In another situation with a young student sealed off in a narcissistic stalemate, the same function is fulfilled by the word "band," which comes to the fore in grandiose contexts of "presidential" ambitions and projects. The term "band" is extraneous to the discourse which again resonates, not in association with "bandits" but rather in the English sense of a group of musicians, which opens the way to the plural.

For the identification and decoding of cryptic messages, the word is often the message, the precious go-between.

The mechanisms of condensation in the word which operate in the analytic dialogue recall the multiple code theory and the referential process of Wilma Bucci (2001, 2009) who describes the wide spectrum of degrees of integration between cognitive and emotional processes. Bucci believes that emotional disturbances are determined by dissociation and distortion between the sub-symbolic experience of the basal affective nucleus and some of the symbolic representations related to the source from which the suffering arises. Listening to the intersubjective communication in the session can detect the reproduction of that generative matrix from which the patient's subjective experience emerges.

Referential Activity is a method for analysing language which identifies and measures active and direct connections between mental representations and words: it is high when it captures a language with qualities of immediacy which mirror a vivid, detailed, and immediate experience; it is low when the language is generic, abstract, and vague.

Power of the "magic" word

The word that is listened to can open worlds: in the history of culture we know that magical formulae have been regarded as keys to open treasure chambers or to bring about magical transformations. We may wonder what this power of the word consists of, given that it is often split off from its meaning, as happens even today in our everyday life when we are lost in the forest of passwords that we need to access our various forms of communication. A word sometimes opens worlds: *Open sesame* (Ferruta 2018).[4]

"Talking cure" is the expression which appears for the first time in Freud's writings as a name for psychoanalytic therapy, and it is remarkable for being a formula enunciated in English and not in German.

"Talking cure" is the expression contained in *Studies on Hysteria* (1892–1895), featuring in the case study of Anna O who, in the acute phase of her psychic suffering, spoke only English. "She aptly described this procedure, speaking seriously, as a 'talking cure,' while she referred to it jokingly as 'chimney-sweeping'" (Freud 1895, p. 30). It is the patient's word, representing not only a concept but also an affect. Indeed, in the *Preliminary Communication* to the *Studies on Hysteria* the question of affect is presented by Freud as fundamental:

> each individual hysterical symptom immediately and permanently disappeared when we had succeeded in bringing clearly to light the memory of the event by which it was provoked and in arousing its accompanying affect, and when the patient had described that event in the greatest possible detail and had put the affect into words.
>
> (Freud 1895, p. 6)

So we can see Freud writing about a *talking cure* not because he had found a German expression capable of describing the therapeutic experience, but because it was a word created by the patient as bearer of a concept and an affect, a word that conveyed a special experience of the patient's, alien to the emotional events of everyday German life, one requiring another voice, another sound, a particular degree of otherness. This was true for Anna O, but probably also for Freud who, in the expression created by the patient, detects the trace of what had been, for her, a discovery about the emotional experience she was living through and, for the therapist, the discovery of a treatment with absolutely novel features that needed to be identified in another language, English, which at that time was certainly not the "common ground" of science and international exchange that it is today.

This detail, linked to the birth of psychoanalysis, prompts a reflection on the power of the word in itself, split off from a meaningful context and a narrative content, like a magic formula, a recurring element in the history of civilisations.

In fables, myths, and riddles the protagonists go in search of the word that has the power to open locked doors, to gain entry to unknown territories, to defeat hugely powerful enemies, to undo paralysing enchantments just like the hysterical paralysis of Anna O.

One example stands for them all: *Open sesame*, a formula known all over the world and in all languages, which has preserved its enigmatic character even though explanations have been sought in the Kabbalah and elsewhere, and well illustrates the power of an apparently simple word, the name of a plant or seed,[5] which unlocks isolated places and fortresses, the rationalising barriers that prevent meeting, communication, sexual rapport.

The phrase appears for the first time in the translation of *A Thousand and One Nights* by Antoine Galland, written between 1704 and 1717, as "*sésame, ouvre-toi*"; in the story, Ali Baba hears the leader of the 40 thieves shout "Open sesame!" and sees a cave entrance open, revealing an enormous quantity of treasure; he uses the same formula to get in and take possession of it. Ali Baba's brother also goes to the cave but, once inside, he forgets the formula and remains trapped in the cave where he is found by the thieves and killed.

The power of the word seems to be connected to something that requires violation without violence, the chance to take possession of the treasures hidden in the cave of the unconscious, bypassing the boundaries of logic or action, using a different mode. Bion's words in *The Grid* come to mind, when he talks about the robbers of royal tombs who "demonstrated the power of gain, and we should perhaps accord them a high position in the Pantheon of Scientific Fame as the forerunners of Science in the domain more usually left in the possession of Magic, Religion and the Dead" (Bion 1977). Perhaps the word in itself, with its evocative power out of logical context, enables us to reach inaccessible places in the unconscious, to comprehend aspects of life and the world that have not yet been reached with the sword of action or the logic of reason.

What is the power of the word in psychoanalysis, in this special *talking cure*? Is the therapeutic factor in interpretation derived from its content, which puts a split-off or repressed content into words so that it finds access to and a home in the mind of the patient, who thus achieves an insight and an awareness of their own psychic history by means of a more complete, deeper narrative? Or is the therapeutic factor the finding of linguistic symbols for concrete sensations and experiences (beta elements), symbols which enable these experiences to become part of the patient's subjective world and transform them into alpha elements that can enlighten, enrich, and inhabit the patient in a tolerable way that is compatible with other representations, as Bion claims? Or is the correspondence of the interpretation with the events of the patient's psychic history not important, just as the integration of never-alphabetised experiences which come to form part of their internal world does not constitute a therapeutic aspect? Is the relationship the only thing that matters? ... a new experience which makes use of verbal and non-verbal communications made by symbols that are not only verbal but conveyed by signs, signals, waves ...

In psychoanalytic therapy and in all psychotherapies, we need to acknowledge the *centrality of communication in words*: even when the relational exchange between patient and analyst privileges other, very primary levels of communication, if we are to make progress we must still take off in the spaceship of the word. In the past 20 years psychoanalytic research has concentrated on the first verbal and non-verbal exchanges between infant and caregiver and illuminated the importance of non-verbal communications linked to profound emotional experiences in the session (Schore 1994); the dimension of the affects as the foundation of all mental and language development (Panksepp and Biven 2012); and the various levels of sub-symbolic states (Bucci 2009). Some time ago Anne Alvarez (2012) drew attention to the importance of agency in children, their vital need to operate as active subjects in the world and not feel that they are only the object of communications that give back projections which are not recognised as expressions in their own right. Sometimes the analyst's communications, which intend to give back the child's projections, merely end up transmitting the activity of signification as expressed only in the analyst's voice. Very often, with severe cases, the first meeting and the early phases of therapy happen in an area where there is a search for – to use the words of Alvarez – a "thinking heart": that is, a lump, a nucleus of affects that are trying to take shape thanks to someone's interest in their presence/ existence, in the perceived possibility of being agents in a relationship. Studies by many Italian psychoanalysts have gone in this direction, anticipating research of this kind: Antonio di Benedetto's (2000) musical listening, attending to what is "before the word"; Agostino Racalbuto's (1994) integrated intervention on several levels "between saying and doing"; Mauro Mancia's (2004) "feeling words" as perceptible sound and rhythm, even before birth; the detailed investigations by Petrella (2018) and Barale (2008) into the musical dimension of communication. But even when we are exploring these precious levels of meeting and of relational communication, the word manifests its fundamental power as a means of transportation and transformation.

Clinical work, as in the case that inaugurates the history of psychoanalysis which I recalled at the start, that of Anna O, helps us to understand and better describe this *mysterious power of the word*. Sometimes during a session an unusual word uttered by the patient, the content of which is not in itself especially significant, strikes the analyst and catches her attention, enabling a process of analysis to begin, a communication that opens worlds just like an "open sesame." I shall give just one example because the interest in this phenomenon is qualitative rather than quantitative. I present the case of a woman aged about 35 who, though gifted (beautiful, intelligent, cultivated, capable), is blocked in her professional and affective life: every significant development gets mired in panic attacks and rage that keep her in an eternal state of stand-by, endlessly on the brink of a new existence. In her analytic sessions too she repeats the experience of not being able to get herself moving towards her desired goals (steady employment instead of temporary contracts, one lasting relationship instead of intermittent ones, a family, children, etc.). In one session, at the end of a sentence about a sister with whom she has broken off relations, and who, despite sharing the same upbringing, has been able to have a partner and children, the patient says, "But she's *avulsed!*" I am struck by the term because it is unusual and not very appropriate for describing a personal situation. In a moment my free-floating attention brings to my mind's eye the image of a basket I had seen in Portugal in a small souvenir shop, with a label on it saying "*Avulsos.*" It contained those polished and decorated ceramic tiles, mostly white and blue, thrown out, then recovered from demolition sites and gathered together, which had once been part of large compositions that decorated the walls of rooms with geometric patterns or scenes from everyday life (hunting, cooking, going for walks: *azulejos*, from the Arabic "*al zulaiga*," a small polished stone) and finally sold as souvenirs. Though it is of Latin origin, the word *avulso* is widely used in Portuguese to indicate something separated by force from a context it belongs to: it contains themes of both union and separation, something detached and independent which at the same time remains part of a whole, containing traces of it; parts of the overall design, for example.[6]

The patient and I work together on this, freely associating: it is something decoupled from both logical and affective links, and is able to rise to the surface of consciousness the way a bubble rises from the depths of the sea; something from the depths that floats using its intrinsic force in spite of the bonds that were holding it under. The word enables us to grasp the fact that the affective bond with something primal is so intrinsic that it outlasts attempts at separation, as if baked on like a design on the tiles: it is both link and isolation, belonging and solitude.

What I find it interesting to highlight is the power of the word, in the sense that a word packed with affects that weigh everything down is able to make this collection of Blegerian ambiguities (Bleger 1967) float: so it seems impossible to apply the classical schema of repressed contents/defences, or the narrative schema which metabolises something raw and renders it introjectible. The word condenses, transports, exceeds, reaches, and opens unconscious worlds that discourse, logic, and sensation would not reach. It both violates and opens, like the tomb robbers, like the 40 thieves.

A word sometimes has a transporting and transforming force, bringing to light a binding nucleus in which contents and affects are intrinsically linked as in the words of poetry: "*avulsed*" transports to the surface of consciousness both the content of the desire for separation and the effect of a link that is impossible to forget, soldered by fire. The word *avulsed* brings into the interaction of the session not the cognitive dimension or even the new reparative experience formed by the relationship with the analyst, but a word that penetrates without immediately activating the bulwarks of the defences, and preserves the character, colours, and qualities of the unique experience linked to the subject's life. It does not replace it with the new analytic experience, casting aside what has been lived, the personal history to which the subject is intrinsically tied and which constitutes him. It unites particular and universal, as certain dream images do. When the analyst's listening catches these emergings in a session, something is achieved which allows us, together with the patient, to open inaccessible worlds without destroying them and without remaining imprisoned: *open sesame.*

The power of the word in analysis is this force which unites concepts, affects, and sensations: when it emerges from the depths of the unconscious it transports something that is the essence of psychoanalysis, this integrity of experience that unites content, affect, sense. *"Avulsed"* opens up the encounter because it does not address the cognitive logic of the infantile history (fusion with the mother), nor the lilting lullaby of nostalgia/*saudade* relived in the session, nor the sonic impact of an excess of consonants – rare in the neo-Latin languages – but condenses, reaching worlds and opening them. Paradoxically, the clinical example reported with *castoff*, which can mean "uprooted," invites me to reflect on the concept of the object's integrity proposed by Bollas: *avulsed* unites many aspects in one word that simultaneously address senses, mind, and heart. Almost always, as in the case of Anna O, the key words that open worlds are offered by the patient herself: we need to refine our ability to catch them with an analytic listening that does not follow logic, guidelines, or protocol, but the unconscious, as Ali Baba does and his brother does not.

Bollas says,

> I think there is a link between language, between speaking and *internal inspiration*. Whatever one's intuition is, one does not ultimately know what one thinks until one speaks, and therefore interpretation creates perspectives that are intimately linked with the unconscious work taking place inside.
>
> (Molino 1997, p. 191)

According to Bollas, emotional experiences are linked to the objects that set them in motion. We construct our personal language via the understanding of forms, configuring our life via the choice of objects that have completeness. The integrity of an experience has the potential to initiate evocative processes: paradoxically, the word *avulsed* picked up by the analyst represents an experience that has its own integrity linked to creative/integrating activity of the subject's unconscious aspects. They function as evocative objects which activate the processes of subjectivating those creations (stories, drawings, music) that have their own integrity of vital, dynamic, unitary functioning and so can be used for processes of re-creation by the subject, who continually assimilates and reorganises new experiences, drawing on an unconscious legacy that is able to emerge. The word is not just a container for the subject's projections, but has its own distinct structure, its own completeness that renders it into a dynamic and efficacious unity, like the *avulsed* tile. When the subject uses it to elaborate and articulate the self, it comes into contact with the completeness of the experience that has its own autonomous life, what we regard as "beauty."

The importance of the word in analysis, alongside discursive interpretation, lies both in this potential for evoking experiences with whole objects and in the direct connection with unitary psychosomatic functioning, as happens in poetry, where the word simultaneously transmits sense, affect, and concept without privileging the cognitive logic of instruction.

This feeling and integration require an experience of the psyche-soma as unitary functioning, an integration which begins to be formed in the first months of life in an experience offered by the maternal caregiving that is provided as a continuity with the child's body. Winnicott talks about a *handling* which fosters this process of the mind's emergence from the body and a feeling that the body is part of a Self that is seated in the body. If, on the contrary, it happens that the mind directs the body as an element which has been differentiated too quickly or too soon, a false self may intervene and there may be depersonalisation and psychosomatic distur-bances as a defence against the loss of unity.

In these cases the use of language risks accentuating the loss of integration, re-iterating a domination of the mind over the body instead of a continuous and fluid passing between the two. Winnicott highlights the fact that the installation of the psyche in the body requires a continuous experience of passing between moments of integration under the Ego's guidance and moments of disintegration and trusting dependency on the other person, especially in periods when new abilities to face the world are being developed (from 2 to 5 years and in the prepubertal period, from 12 to 14). The recovery of a language function as an element of psycho-corporeal inte-gration happens through immersion in intense sensations that traverse this distance. A present-day medical and pedagogic tendency to provide a series of behavioural prescriptions through language ends up accentuating this distance and becomes an element of depersonalisation. The word ends up losing its contact with the body and arrives at the body as a guide that accentuates its extraneousness.

Instead we can learn from what happens with rhyme in poetry: Mario Fubini, a literary scholar commenting on Dante and the tradition of *terza rima* in Italian po-etry, highlighted the lifegiving and restructuring potency of new meaning achieved by the alternating rhyme of *terza rima*, when two words that have never encoun-tered each other before are brought together, causing surprise and emotion, thereby regaining body and meaning.

A significant example is given by the lines describing the suicide of Pier Delle Vigne in Canto XIII of the *Inferno* where the rhyme brings together the dryness of the "*sterpi*" (stocks) which the suicides have turned into and the "*serpi*" (serpents), chthonic animals representing life alongside death in the symbols of medicine, ever since Asclepius:

> When it had become dark with blood, it began again to cry, Why dost thou tear me? Hast thou not any spirit of pity? Men we were, and now we are become stocks; truly thy hand ought to be more pitiful had we been the souls of serpents.
>
> (XIII, 34–40, 1891, p. 62)[7]

The contemporary poet Patrizia Valduga has written a love poem in *terza rima*, *La tentazione* [Temptation], and at the moment when her desire reveals itself in the display of a body being impudently shown off, a rhyme unites the words "*sogno*" (dream) and "*vergogno*" (I am ashamed), communicating the irresistible need to condense desire and body into a single revelation with the shame from which the dream offers shelter: "Under my humble sky, / like a dream dreamt inside a dream, / I cover my face with a veil / now because I am ashamed of many things"[8] (Valduga 1977, pp. 165–166).

Sometimes language loses its function as a messenger between mind and body, between conscious and unconscious, is weakened and diminished when it becomes taught and teaching speech. So it must go back to the body and its sensations in order to regain the vital unconscious sap of the evocative poetic word. However, the word always maintains its distinctive performative dimension, even outside the context of the magic formula: the poet changes the use of the word in order to change the world.

The word as a way out of the subject's "enigmatic privacy"

The word offers an experience addressed by one subject to another subject: intimate, unique, and special. This means listening with all one's being, trusting one's experience of things, restoring the word's sensory root, using the "spoken" word to encounter another human being and not to unleash a war of words, nor as a substitute for experience (Ferruta 2010).[9]

In its sensory, affective, and semantic fullness, the word vectorially addressed to another person acts as a bridge between the Sphinx's riddle and the dialect of Athens: "With the word, the infant has found a new transformational object, which facilitates the transition from deep enigmatic privacy towards the culture of the human village" (Bollas 1987, p. 35).[10]

Listening to silence

Silence is someone listening

The analyst's silence in the consulting room has often been the subject of stories told in ironic, paradoxical terms. It is as if the analyst's silence were like that of an inaccessible divinity to whom the analysand has turned for a response or the solution to a riddle, like an oracle that remains silent and inscrutable. This conception mirrors an area of analysis that is no longer widely practised. Instead psychoanalysis has advanced by developing a relational, interactive, intersubjective dimension in which the psychoanalytic process unfolds through the meeting between the unconsciouses of two committed subjects, to the point where analysts not only intervene frequently, but sometimes go further, talk about themselves and their emotions, "out" themselves ... And the patients end up hearing too many voices: those of persecutors or authority figures, not internalised but projected outwards; and others too ...

Let us instead try and listen to some "voices of the silence" which emerge during analysis.

Freud (1912) talks about the mental position of the analyst, using the metaphor of the opaque mirror which shows the analysand only what is shown to it: he listens with his unconscious like a telephone receiver ready to receive the patient's communications without introducing his own interferences, listening to the other openly, without prejudices, like a receptive organ. These assertions by Freud are the foundation of psychoanalysis as space and time for listening to what comes from elsewhere: "He should simply listen, and not bother about whether he is keeping anything in mind" (Freud 1912, p. 112).

In poetic essays Enzo Morpurgo (1998) has described this analytic quality of making silence away from the world's uproar, even though he is a psychoanalyst dedicated to promoting the social dimension of psychoanalysis, opening a clinic for psychoanalytic psychotherapy in the bustling Milanese district of Niguarda, and also studying the philosophical dimension of psychoanalytic knowledge, as well as poetry where the written word is everything. Morpurgo sharply differentiates social dialogue, focused on ordinary everyday interaction – which he considers pathogenic – from analytic dialogue, which gives space for whatever has no audience in everyday social existence. Analytic dialogue stays open to listening to the other's suffering as the bringer of a double need: to put what is bad into the other and to present themselves as someone other than their usual self.[11]

The analyst offers a wide unprejudiced listening to help the patient get in touch with the voices inside, with what comes from somewhere else but is suffocated, overwhelmed by internal and external encumbrances, with the aim of going on to feel direct, personal experiences, and to find words for communicating them.

The analyst's listening to the silence in the session must symmetrically refine the analysand's capacity for listening to the emotions of their private life, which their primary objects may have been deaf to, inducing a kind of mutism, an absence of subjectivated interactions in the relational field. We know that this deafness results in mutism, a difficulty in giving voice to experiences that a primary object was deaf to, as if they did not exist, and which the analyst must listen to for the first time, without being dazzled by other more obvious, "visible" elements in the patient's history. I recall a Sicilian patient who came to Milan for doctoral research at the university and who, until the first snowfall of the year, had only known snow as an image in photographs. He was amazed to find that the snow made a sound, that faint noise as the crystalline flakes yielded under the pressure of his footsteps. The blinding whiteness of the snow can wipe out other sensations, for example, the pressure one's foot exerts on the snow, the force of a living presence not "'whited out'" or frozen by the predominance of other senses (sight, touch) over the sense of hearing. The snow has a voice, a sound, it is not only a visual and tactile experience, but also a sonic one. I similarly recall a deeply moving video account made by a patient who had been deaf from birth and was given a cochlear implant by Professor Gregorio Babighian, a Tunisian ENT surgeon who used to go back to his native region in the desert to hear voices that make themselves felt in the silence. In his video the patient talked about waking up from the implant operation: the first sound he heard was the lunch trolley clattering as the orderlies wheeled it around the ward. Among the unknown sounds he had not expected was the surprising crunch of dry leaves during his first walk in the park, another experience of the subject's "force," an experience now undergone with a sonic accompaniment, unlike anything he had ever known.

In Henckel's film *The Lives of Others* (2006), the listening to other people's voices is carried out by the diligently indifferent Stasi agent in the silence of the attic where he hides to perform his persecutory monitoring of the tenants on behalf of the secret police. Little by little it generates an openness to other worlds within his private hearing so that, in the end, he listens to his own voice too, which until that moment had remained mute. And lastly, we cannot be silent about the extraordinary listening of Alan Turing, breaker of the Enigma code, to whom we are greatly indebted for our survival and liberty, who was so committed and skilful as he listened with intelligence and passion to the Third Reich's secret code. In his difference from others, Turing did not find space for his own personal, intimate secret to be listened to, but was convicted of homosexuality, then a crime in Britain, and forced to choose between prison and chemical castration. He chose the latter but after two years took his own life, biting into an apple impregnated with cyanide. No one had listened to his voice, mechanically recorded in a statement which was officially ordered to be deleted. In the same way, seven Trappist monks from the abbey of Tibhirine had their "tongues cut out" during the conflict between Moslems and Christians in Algeria. They were killed by religious fanaticism because in the hostel at their silent monastic community they accommodated and listened to something that was different.[12]

So does silence mean listening that creates a space of silence in ourselves, or producing a silence by keeping other people quiet? Today many therapies and educational services are directed to at quietening the voices of suffering, lack, absence, or difference (Petrella 1998). "'Silencers'" are offered and sought in the form of food, drugs, or detailed instructions to follow well-trodden paths: stoppers used like the baby's dummies that Winnicott (1968) jokingly called "passifiers" instead of "pacifiers" in a letter to Renata Gaddini which she quoted in a fine paper of her own on "The precursors of the object and of transitional phenomena."[13] Instead we should offer a listening that gives space and time so that, as Masud Khan (1979, p. 19) says, "the innate biological capacities can be realised in a personalised psychic space."

I suggest we think about silence in analysis as the way of reaching that which is not immediately perceptible, and about the analyst as what Bollas (1999) calls a talking canvas, a listening that gives a voice and a word for constructing the subject who is other-than-oneself. The fact that the analyst does not answer the patient's questions may be hard for those outside the analytic sphere to understand. I will dwell briefly on two areas in particular that are too often silenced: *zones of silence* and *sibling bonds*.

Zones of silence: Denied suffering

Sometimes we come across signs telling us that we are entering zones of silence where the use of a car horn or other noise-making devices is prohibited, usually near hospitals or care homes. The overt intention is not to disturb ill people who need rest and tranquillity. But this request can also be understood as intended to silence human suffering, to avoid it, to act as if it wasn't there. The link with the suffering of the other person symbolically represents the suffering that is deposited in everyone's heart as an inevitable aspect of being human, through the existence of the body and the transient relationship with other people, who are mortal.

When psychoanalysis appeared as a discipline in the early twentieth century, one zone of silence, avoided and concealed in hysterical symptoms, was sexuality. Today, with the societal changes that have happened and are still in progress, we can ask ourselves what the silent zones are, the areas being kept quiet, which the patient who comes to analysis is asking to give a voice.

The narcissistic pathologies are multiplying, with the presence and reality of the other-than-oneself becoming a cause of suffering – in other words, insufferable – and not playing a part in the construction of the subject. Kaës (2008) has shown that many individual and societal problems are connected to the construction of nega-tory narcissistic "deals" based on denial of the link that the individual personality needs with the other. Shush! The negatory alliance involves whatever needs the other's cooperation in order to be cancelled, a cooperation that is necessary if the link is to be maintained in a complementarity of interests. The negatory alliance is a meta-defence that creates zones of silence, pockets of intoxication that keep a subject outside both his own story and the other's.

We find an example of this in Elie Wiesel's book *Night* (1958) set in the village of Sighet, where Wiesel himself lived as a boy. It recounts the return of Moshe, the first resident to be deported, simply because he was a foreigner, but who survived a mass execution under a pile of corpses. Moshe tries to explain to the other villag-ers what has happened and is about to happen, but no one listens. He is unable to establish that link with a live and healthy sociality that may aid survival:

> You can't understand. I have been saved miraculously. I managed to get back here. Where did I get the strength from? I wanted to come back to Sighet to tell you the story of my death. So that you could prepare yourselves while there was still time. To live? I don't attach any importance to my life any more. I'm alone. No, I wanted to come back, and to warn you. And see how it is, no one will listen to me.
>
> (Wiesel 1958)

Narcissism as an illness built on the silence of the link with the other that is crucial in constituting the subject, and on the extraneousness of illness and death, which "'only happen to other people'"!

Philìa: A sibling bond

Psychoanalysis has contributed to making everyone aware, even in the shared culture of non-specialists, of the strength and importance of the familial bonds that unite parents and children. The Oedipus complex and consequent rivalry with the parents, the desired and condemned incest, and transgenerational violence are widely known across society and not silenced. Rivalry in general with the parents is acknowledged and rendered benign by developing the processes of identification and becoming parents and procreators in our own turn.

By contrast, silence seems to be imposed on the sibling bond which unites human beings of the same generation and requires a place to be left for the other even when they do not hold a position of generational or social authority. The other, the sibling, seems to be a silenced dimension, one exposed to violation, not safeguarded by the laws of the *polis*.

In her paper presented at the 2012 Congress of the Italian Psychoanalytic Society in Rome on "Psychic Reality and Social Rules," Silvana Borutti spoke about *philìa* as a sibling bond which is constitutive of the subject but is often denied for narcissistic reasons, the refusal to make room for the other in a bond built on reciprocity rather than a transgenerational hierarchy.

Borutti says,

If we do not understand what I would call the *primal rule* – that is, the need to acknowledge our primally heterological constitution, through which relationship does not supervene to unite monadic subjectivities but is constitutive of subjectivity itself – then rules in general are not understood, the point of them is not understood. The Greeks have a fundamental word/concept for this condition of primal incompleteness and recognition of the other in oneself: not *eros* but *philìa*. By means of this concept they come to think about the other in the constituting of the subject.

(Borutti 2012, p. 21)

Borutti thinks of Antigone not as a character who gives priority to the blood-tie with her unburied brother Polyneices, but as someone who asserts the value and potency of *philìa*, of the law based on the incompleteness of the subject and its constitution which is primally bound to the other-than-oneself.

According to Borutti, Antigone's invoking of the sibling bond in the form of the blood-tie would plunge this bond back into silence and put trust only in the law written in the body and dispensing with the word. This means listening to the other even when one has no position of authority, because the other is a fundamental element of shared existence: on the one hand, it limits individual freedom but, on the other, broadens it to include what we do not know of ourselves or of what we will become (Bollas 1987).

Reciprocity is a dimension that includes difference and mirroring, the ability to move back and forth in both directions, between self and other, without getting lost. A bridge must be crossed (Ferruta 2008) between Asia and Europe, over a Hellespont crossed many times before with shipwrecks and drownings, as narrated in the myth of Hero and Leander,[14] a truly dynamic psychoanalysis that can unite pleasure in the encounter with the other and sufficient cohesion of the self.

This is why analytic work can be classed among the realms of the intermediate, like art and play: an activity that continually transforms silence into co-constructed word, the fruit of the encounter (Ferro 2007), into an intersubjective analytic third (Ogden 2009) who takes over the word. The words that are formed in analysis are what did not exist previously, like the word in poetry, the note in music, or the painter's brushstroke.

This is something that comes into being in the listening of someone who is able to silence their own narcissism in order to meet the other and listen to the unknown voice, never heard before, the sound of the snow and leaves underfoot, the timbre of *The Magic Flute* felt in Peter Brook's production at the Teatro Strehler in Milan; a single note vibrating on the triangle, a single note that lights up and widens the universe. In an interview given at the premiere of *The Magic Flute*, Brook (2010) observes,

> Today we try to explain everything, to make everything clear: and yet the strength of what we call poetry, the energy of what we call music, lies in their ability to surpass that limit since they begin in that precise moment when rational explanation can go no further.

Analysis opens by listening to those creative notes that emerge from a meeting, as explanations and prescriptions are diminished, making space for sound, the movement of the dance, the evocative word of poetry.

The frail instrument represented by a triangle, hanging in mid-air, which then vanishes in the finale of the drama, is magical because it can make the categories of pedagogy disappear, and allows the characters to present themselves as bearers of an essentiality, that of the soul's music which resonates internally with a few, equally essential notes: wisdom, love, friendship, and no others. This *flute/triangle* is an open space, free of encumbrances, like the mind of an analyst who is open to the meeting with an unknown subject. An analyst who listens to the crunching of the snow and leaves under the feet of a subject moving in the world, one who is not immobilised in a diagnosis or in a transferential relationship that compulsively repeats. It requires the silence of someone who is listening.

An envelope of words: the psychic skin

The skin as a psychic function that holds the self together

The psychoanalyst who has most engaged with the psychic function of the skin is Didier Anzieu who wrote beautifully about it in a fundamental text, *Le Moi-peau* [*The Skin-Ego*] (1985). Anzieu is also an author much concerned with the group psyche, having conducted group therapies and worked out a theory of the psychic apparatus which includes the group dimension within the functioning of the individual. In his clinical experience and his theorising he draws attention to how the psychic skin contains multiple fragments of experience which need a cohering function so that the subject can operate as a unit and communicate with others.

Besides the function of the skin, Anzieu (1990) describes how, earlier still, the selectively permeable membrane surrounds the cell and maintains an electrochemical gradient between internal and external: "asymmetry thus appears to be coextensive with life." Anzieu holds that the basic psychic envelope is tactile, permitting simultaneous sensory experiences of touch and feeling touched, as the first basis for differentiation between self and other. He dwells at length on the pathology of the container, which plays a role not only as a passive receiver of images, emotions, and sensations from the child but also, by means of subjective mechanisms, as an active transformer. The function of the receptive and active receiver may be deficient, either because it is lacking, leaving the individual in an undifferentiated state, or because the envelope has been formed but is punctuated by holes which cause an internal emptying out of everything that goes into creating the subject's strength, a kind of narcissistic haemorrhage: all the resources seem to come from outside.

Another psychoanalyst, Eugenio Gaddini, in collaboration with the paediatrician, child neuropsychiatrist, and psychoanalyst Renata Gaddini De Benedetti, has made a detailed study of the earliest areas of the child's psychic development, based on a body–mind continuum set-up by the gradual organising of a first sense of self.[15] After birth, the environment should be capable of providing that stable boundary which the infant has lost on emerging from the experience of the uterine container: primary maternal care (*holding* and *handling*) enables the child to pass gradually from a fragmentary condition of non-integration to a first unitary psychic organisation. Eugenio Gaddini identified the moment when the child starts to draw circular forms instead of simple scribbles as manifesting the first perception of the self as a unitary subject with boundaries, distinct from the environment in which it is immersed, thanks to an envelope which simultaneously gives it shape, protects it, and enables it to communicate with other people ("The Mask and the Circle," 1985). The Gaddinis describe a skin disease of the first months of life, at around six months, atopic dermatitis, as one of the syndromes that manifest themselves at a specific time, an expression of difficulty in the process of forming the psychic skin as a container for the self. The subject has not been helped by that maternal handling that Winnicott talks about: that is, the caregiver's ability to enable a continuity to be felt between the other's touch and the psychosomatic envelope, until the moment when this continuity of touch becomes proprioception of self and of one's own boundaries: "The defence of dermatitis makes manifest the fact that the boundary of one's own skin (of the separate self) is not able to 'hold' and protect what it contains (in fact, the physical treatment of dermatitis guarantees constant contact)" (Gaddini E. 1980, p. 484).[16]

Any psychic function develops with the support of a bodily function, whose operation is transposed onto the mental plane. The skin (surface of the body) and the brain (surface of the nervous system) have the same embryonic structure, the ectoderm. The psyche—skin relationship concerns formations that are developed in the earliest period of life, at the origin of the psychic apparatus, when the processes of self-containment are activated, profoundly involving the cohesion of the parts that constitute the self and the relation of the individual to the other-than-self. The skin provides the representations that constitute the Ego and its functions.[17]

From a psychological viewpoint, we can think of the skin as an organ of the individual that carries out structurally fundamental functions, and not think only of the skin's metaphorical significance. We can think of the skin as an envelope containing the self and as a limit marking the boundary between self and other. The distance is not only the one that is needed so that our visual field can have a perception of the other-than-self, but is also a distance which signifies the perception of oneself as a subject different from another. (Consider, by contrast, those with psychotic pathologies who tend towards an unsustainable closeness or isolate themselves in a rigid rejection of the other, shutting themselves away in a room.)

The integrity of the container-skin does not only have the symbolic value of marking the boundaries between self and other, but also performs the role of transformative filter which allows someone to come close to the other without finding it too painful, as when we have a wound or an abrasion, or to feel pleasure or unpleasure depending on the quality of the experience that the other is offering. Thus, following Anzieu, the skin carries out the function of container, barrier, filter, mirror (sack, shield, sieve, screen).

I recall the case of a young man who shut himself away in his room, refusing all contact, and experienced a vulnerability and extreme psychic permeability to the stimuli from the environment, which were desired but perceived as invasive and capable of altering him. One of the first times he was able to leave his isolation and go to the seaside with a friend, he put on two wetsuits to go into the water, with the multiple aim of keeping his haemorrhaging sensations together, protecting him from abuse by the cold extraneousness of not-me reality, and enabling him to be with others and communicate what he had perceived through his skin.

How much otherness can a subject integrate within the boundaries of the self without being broken? The skin is an organ that holds together and communicates with the other-than-self: contact with the other-than-self provides constant progressive perceptions of one's own uniqueness. Think of neonates who want to be picked up and held, or who were previously being swaddled, who start to turn towards the transitional objects which are becoming their possession by contact with the skin: all experiences that enable them to perceive the boundaries of the self as an element giving form to the Skin-Ego, so that they can say, *I am*. The mother who envelops the baby with her caregiving is internalised little by little and ensures the sense of the Self's continuity. Think of dropouts who isolate themselves, sleeping rough under bridges and in doorways, refusing contact with others while covering themselves up even in high summer, as a stand-in for that mental function of the Skin-Ego which has perhaps not been able to develop adequately. Contact with the skin of the other-than-self contributes to the construction and structuring of the subject.

The skin as a psychic function that communicates with the other-than-self

Contact with the other is necessary not only for building the integrity of the self, the Skin-Ego envelope, but also for establishing currents of communication with the not-me. The pores of the skin are a continuous channel of communication, an open window onto desired and needed otherness. I recall the case of a young man who sweated so profusely in the consulting room that he left a mark like a shroud on the cover of the couch. He was coming for treatment because of difficulties in relating to other people, his struggle to get along with his peers, troubled by contradictory desires for closeness and differentiation. To me, the sweat immediately seemed to manifest a desire to communicate with the analyst, against himself and in spite of everything, to leave a trace of himself in the session.

In summary, Anzieu describes *nine functions of the Skin-Ego* (Anzieu 1985, pp. 98–106):

- support (holding)
- container (handling)
- para-excitation
- individuation
- intersensoriality
- sexual excitation
- libidinal recharging of the psychic functions
- registering tactile sensory traces
- self-destruction along the lines of autoimmune disease.

As we reflect on the psychic function of this bodily organ composed by the skin, we can make a first hypothesis along the way: one about breaks in the envelope, which concern the relationship with the other-than-self and present features that crack the cohesion of the self, threaten it, put it to the test. We can try to understand whether these cracks, lesions, disturbances of the skin envelope affect certain subjects more frequently than others. Such subjects often have a great desire for encounters and exchanges with other people and from the outset, for the most part unconsciously, they test the firmness of the self's container. They are subjects characterised by an insufficient experience of the transitional area, either because of a superabundant desire or a kind of temporal short-circuit which abbreviates the time needed for metabolising experiences that come from the other-than-self. We know that many dermatological disturbances are to do with metabolic dysfunctions and particularly intense immune reactions: we could see the intensely desired other-than-self as having not been adequately digested and metabolised, and being expelled into the aspects of the organism that the subject cannot tolerate. The metabolising of other-ness takes time that is often short-circuited, underestimating its dissimilarity to the somatopsychic organism which is taking in the unfamiliar "food," just as in the experience of an encounter with a stranger, even though it is strongly desired and valued. Afflictions of the skin in subjects who desire encounters with other people often leave them profoundly frustrated and saddened by this difficulty. Some dermatological manifestations are characterised by expelling onto the level of the skin something that has nowhere else to go and finally surfaces, becoming visible to other people.

Here we are touching on other features present, especially in subjects exposed to problems with their skin: a withheld and controlled aggressiveness that finds no other outlet such as physiological evacuation or the evacuation of tension through dialogue with others or in action, such as sport. Emotions that one is ashamed of and would rather hide surface via the skin, coming through and being seen against the subject's conscious wishes: the blush of desire, the pallor of fear, the hair standing on end in the cold of loneliness. The skin speaks of a sensitive self that one would rather conceal, hide away, keep safe from exposure to sarcasm, offence, the other's gaze. The skin reminds us of our vulnerability, our nakedness without excessive defences of intellectualisation and distance, as in the first moments of life and in the sexual encounter: without defences other than those formed by the minimal wrapping of the skin that guarantees the self's cohesion, the perception of what is me and what is the other, a subtle boundary on which we meet "I am" and "I love you" and "I hate you." A highly vulnerable boundary that is sometimes defensively thickened to avoid injury, at other times thinned in order to communicate with that which we are not and do not know. We need to develop a relationship that enables us to reappropriate the sensory bases of the psyche.[18]

Immersed in a bath of words

Psychoanalytic practice and infant research agree that the regulation of affects and emotions is a fundamental component in skin disorders, especially systemic ones. At the same time, this psychosomatic functioning which governs the vulnerability of the psyche-soma is constructed on very archaic levels that are hard to reach in a psychotherapeutic relationship. Psychotherapeutic treatment can undoubtedly reach and treat the effects of this somatopsychic malfunctioning: difficulty making relationships with others; depression resulting from a disturbance that has damaged the subject's healthy narcissism; the realisation of how intense a desire is felt for sociability and sharing; sensitivity to interhuman contact.

But the treatment has a very limited ability to reach archaic levels of psychic functioning and to transform them, compared to other psychosomatic disturbances linked to more accessible modes of functioning associated with functions from less early stages (digestive disturbances, migraine, pains caused by bad posture, etc.). Current developments in the theory of the psychic apparatus and of psychoanalytic technique are heading in a hopeful direction because they rely less on verbally interpreting the contents of the relationship between analyst and patient, and more on thinking of the treatment as a relational experience in which what matters are the emotions being felt in the present moment, which allow us to think of the therapy as a new beginning. Balint (1967) spoke of a basic fault which characterises the functioning of certain subjects who need treatment in order to re-experience with a therapist a relationship in which regression is central to the engagement, and the therapist's role is taken for granted like the ground we walk on and the air we breathe. Anzieu (1996) used to rebuild the envelope around the cohesion of the self in the session by providing an envelope of sound, a bath of words in which subjects could immerse themselves, little by little regaining contact with the experience of perceiving boundaries in a way that was not alienating or traumatic. Offering the patient a signifier in these treatments means giving form to a series of disaggregated sensations that start to be unified and play a part in the cohesion of the self: here this function of giving form, acting as a means of demarcation which carries out this function, becomes more important the less it corresponds to a real object (building with Lego, dinosaurs, fantasy animals, etc.). Its elaboration in psychoanalytic care requires work not of interpretation but of construction. The formation of containers is just as important as the formation of contents.

Notes

1 "So I think it becomes essential to try and teach the candidate to learn the patient's language, that particular dialect of theirs, which may be so distant from our own, instead of claiming that they must adjust themselves to ours" (Nissim Momigliano 1992, pp. 75–76).
2 Donnet is referring to the article "On Psychotherapy" (1904) where Freud cites a distinction made by Leonardo da Vinci between painting, which works "by putting on" and sculpture which works "by taking away."
3 Visual perception according to Gestalt is a process that develops by following certain rules for organising the perceived data. For example: *good form* (the perceived structure is always the simplest); *proximity* (the elements are grouped in terms of the distance between them); *likeness* (tendency to group similar elements together); *good continuity* (all the elements are perceived as belonging to a coherent and continuous whole); *figure-ground* (all the parts of an area can be interpreted both as object and as background); etc.
4 This section largely reprises the content of the article: Ferruta A. (2018). Apriti sesamo. Il potere della parola. *Educazione sentimentale* 30, 36–44. Edizioni Franco Angeli.
5 The seeds of the herbaceous sesame plant, originally from India and Africa, given the scientific name *Sesamum indicum*, is a precious source of nutritive elements enclosed in each of their minuscule dimensions. They can be regarded as among the most important seeds for maintaining a good level of health, a major source of calcium. Indeed, 100 g of sesame seeds may contain 800–1000 mg of calcium. In the same quantity of sesame there are about 470 mg of phosphorus, 815 mg of magnesium and 20.1 mg of iron, as well as 18.7 per cent protein. Antioxidant and anti-cancer properties have been attributed to sesame seeds. Their lignan content assists in controlling blood pressure and reducing hypertension. The consumption of sesame seeds may contribute to preventing the formation of plaques on artery walls. Intake of sesame seeds is beneficial for the bones, improves liver function, is effective in removing intestinal worms, reduces rheumatism and joint pain, stimulates the circulation, and contributes to improving the digestion. Sesame oil extracted from the seeds is used in skin care as an aid in invigorating massages.
6 1. Arrancado ou separado à força. 2. Que não faz parte de um todo. 3. Separado, isolado, insulado. 4. Desligado do corpo ou da coleção de que fazia parte; desirmanado. Existem várias aplicações do conceito de avulso. Em um sentido físico, este termo é usado para localizar alguém ou algo fora de contato com outras pessoas ou fatores. Um homem que está trancado em uma cela que só tem uma ventilação para respirar, sem janelas e uma porta blindada que se abre a partir do lado exterior, estão em uma condição de isolamento máximo, um modo avulso máximo de ficar: não pode ver outra pessoa ou falar com ninguém.

7 Da che fatto fu poi di sangue bruno,
   ricominciò a dir: "Perché mi scerpi?
   non hai tu spirto di pietà alcuno?
   Uomini fummo, e or siam fatti sterpi:
   ben dovrebb'esser la tua man più pia,
   se state fossimo anime di serpi." (XIII, 34–40).

8 Sotto il mio umile cielo
   come un sogno sognato dentro un sogno
   ora la faccia mi copro di un velo
   perché di molte cose mi vergogno"

9 The clairvoyant word of Christa Wolf's Cassandra (1983) is not listened to because it lacks an interlocutor in the relational dimension of a potential "we": "… who I am. To see only conquerors in you and not also those who will live. Who must live, so that what we call life can go on. These poor conquerors must go on living for all those they have killed. I say to them: if you can stop conquering. This city of yours will go on existing" (Wolf 1983). "'We' I say, and all We whom I have approached, this remains the thing that troubles me the most. It is much easier to say to the beast Achilles than to this We" (Wolf 1983). [Translated from the Italian versions of the passages from Wolf.]

10 Paul Ricoeur's reflection on "the extension of the semiotic sphere *to the obscure boundaries of the mute desire that precedes language*" (2020, p. 414) is quoted with a comment in the Preface "Paul Ricoeur and Psychoanalysis" by Francesco Barale and in the Afterword "La voie longue 'Autour de la psychanalyse: approdi" by Giuseppe Martini.

11 "While posing the problem of the other used to be philosophically complex for all of us, and equally complex existentially, I believe that this may all change radically when acceptance of the other becomes acceptance of the other's pain and his need to find comfort. I believe that in a couple or a group, the expression of internal malaise creates an image in the listener which substantially destabilises the preconscious idea of the subject's identity in time. I believe that this otherness of the suffering other is the source of the pathogenic character of the response … That the psychoanalyst is in fact the partner in the analytic couple, and is better equipped than the patient's life partner. The analyst, protected by the setting, can face the expression of pain but is also exposed to the temptation to reject it. And perhaps does so using sophisticated theories, such as I have often come across even in writers who theorise about empathy with the patient … In cases like those the analyst uses his theory – whichever it may be – to defend himself rather than more simply but more laboriously, accepting, receiving, and tolerating the patient's pain. Giving the patient and himself all the time needed to understand or even not understand; or to understand and not be able to do anything for the distress or suffering being expressed; because this too means accepting the 'horizon of death' in the session, as a sign of the limit, of the fact that there is no guarantee of success in the psychoanalytic enterprise" (Morpurgo 1998, pp. 202–204).

12 In the words of the leaflet introducing the monastery to its guests, "Guests of the Algerian people, who are almost entirely Moslem, these brothers wish to bear witness that peace between peoples is a gift from God, made for men of every place and every time, and that believers, here and now, should make manifest this inalienable gift, especially through the quality of their mutual respect and the demanding maintenance of a healthy and fertile spiritual competition …. The hostel – or house reserved for guests – belongs to this same vocation of welcome and sharing, listening and praise, silence and unity" (Chenu 1996, pp. 29–30).

13 "What usually happens with dummies, which Winnicott jokingly called 'passifiers' rather than 'pacifiers' (Winnicott 1968) – i.e., they make babies passive instead of peaceful – is that mothers 'shove' them into the child's mouth so that he has no choice but to become quiet … What is completely absent in the dummy technique is the baby's

search, his *movement towards* something … In other words, no credit is given for the child's creative capacity, or for a mouth that can go towards an object with saliva" (Gaddini R. 1970, p. 281).

14 Leander of Abydos in Asia Minor is in love with Hero, priestess of Artemis in the temple of Sestos on the opposite Greek shore. So that they can meet, Leander swims the Hellespont every night guided by the torch that Hero lights on the temple tower. One night the wind blows out the flame and Leander drowns, having lost his point of reference. In her grief, Hero throws herself from the tower into the sea. Their myth is recounted in a poem by Musaeus, VI century CE. Byron swam the Hellespont in order to revive the story of the two lovers.

15 "Psychoanalysis considers the body and the mind as a functioning 'continuum,', the key element of which remains the fact that it is a process in the differentiating of the mental function which runs from body to mind, and yet psychoanalysis studies it in the opposite direction" (Gaddini E., 1980, p. 470).

16 "It seems to me we can say that in general the psycho-physical syndromes of the first eighteen months (and perhaps later, whenever a development is in progress) refer to a pathology of the mind related to detachment and separateness. As a result, they manifest themselves at certain moments of early development when the problem is especially pressing, and – in a sort of concrete, pre-verbal, and pre-symbolic language, which is that of an altered bodily functioning – they express a defensive mental content specific to the moment of mental development in which the problem emerges. A syndrome that only intervenes at around the sixth month of life (on rare occasions a little earlier) is atopic dermatitis. During this period, while detachment and separation of selves are in progress – when, if the relationship with the environment is more or less good enough, a transitional object starts to intervene from the seventh month onwards – the mental difficulty or impossibility of continuing along the line of development may instead be expressed in the form of somatic pathology. In this case, there will be no trace of a transitional object in subsequent months (De Benedetti Gaddini 1974), and the manifest pathology will affect the skin" (Gaddini E. 1980, pp. 483–484).

17 "By Skin Ego I mean a mental image of which the Ego of the child makes use during the early phases of its development to represent itself as an Ego containing psychical contents, on the basis of its experience of the surface of the body" (Anzieu 1985, p. 40).

18 Fundamental concepts for Anzieu (1990, p. 57) are: basic narcissistic security (holding, handling, growing autonomy of the psychic apparatus); shared skin and separation; self-organisation by reciprocal construction of the Ego and the object; contained container.

References

Alighieri, D. (1891). *The Divine Comedy. Volume 1 – Hell*. Translated by Charles Eliot Norton. Kiberside Press, Cambridge.

Alvarez A. (2012). *The Thinking Heart*. Routledge, Hove.

Anzieu D. (1985). *The Skin-Ego*. Yale, New Haven, 1989.

Anzieu D. (1990). *L'epidermide nomade e la pelle psichica*. Raffaello Cortina Editore, Milan, 1992.

Anzieu D. (1994). *Le penser. Du moi-peau au moi-pensant*. Dunod, Paris.

Anzieu D. (1996). I significanti formali e l'Io-pelle. In Anzieu D. et al. *Gli involucri psichici*. Dunod, Milan, 1997.

Aulagnier P. (1975). *The Violence of Interpretation: From Pictogram to Statement*. Brunner-Routledge, Hove, 2001.

Balint M. (1967). *The Basic Fault: Therapeutic Aspects of Regression*. Tavistock, London.

Barale F. and Minazzi V. (2008). Off the Beaten Track: Freud, Sound and Music. Statement of a Problem and Some Historico-Critical Notes. *Int. J. Psycho-Anal.* 89, 937–957.

Bion W. R. (1967). Notes on Memory and Desire. *Psychoanalytic Forum* 2, 271–280.

Bion W. R. (1977). *Two Papers: The Grid and the Cæsura.* Abingdon, Routledge, 2018.

Bleger J. (1967). *Simbiosi e ambiguità.* Libreria Editrice Lauretana, Loreto 1992.

Bollas C. (1987) *The Shadow of the Object: Psychoanalysis of the Unthought Known.* Routledge, Abingdon, 2018.

Bollas C. (1992). *Being a Character.* Routledge, Hove.

Bollas C. (1995). *Cracking up.* Routledge, London.

Bollas C. (1999). *The Mystery of Things.* Routledge, London.

Borutti S. (2012). La *philìa* come regola originaria. Paper presented at the Congress of the Italian Psychoanalytic Society on *Realtà psichica e regole sociali,* Rome.

Brook P. (2010). Interview with ARTE, at the opening night of *Une flute enchantée* (Paris, 10 November 2010, at the Théâtre des Bouffes du Nord).

Bucci W. (2001). Pathways of Emotional Communication. *Psychoanal. Inq.* 21, 1, 40–70.

Bucci W. (2009). Lo spettro dei processi dissociativi. Implicazioni per la relazione terapeutica. In Moccia G. and Solano L. (eds.) *Psicoanalisi e neuroscienze.* Angeli, Milan.

Chenu B. (eds.) (1996). *Più forti dell'odio.* Piemme, Casale Monferrato.

Chodorow N. (2012). Analytic Listening and the Five Senses: Introduction. *JAPA* 60, 4, 747–758.

Di Benedetto A. (2000). *Prima della parola. L'ascolto psicoanalitico del non detto attraverso le forme dell'arte.* Angeli, Milan.

Donnet J.L. (2008). De l'attention en egal suspens à l'écoute métapsychologique. www. spp. asso.fr/textes/textes-et-conferences/reflexions-de-psychanalystes-2.

Faimberg H. (1981). "'Listening to Listening: An Approach to the Study of Narcissistic Resistances.'" In *The Telescoping of Generations: Listening to the Narcissistic Links Between Generations.* Routledge, Hove.

Faimberg H. (2005). *The Telescoping of Generations: Listening to the Narcissistic Links between Generations.* Routledge, London and New York.

Ferro A. (2007). *Avoiding Emotions, Living Emotions.* Routledge, Hove, 2011.

Ferruta A. (2008). *Crossing the Bridge.* Identità e cambiamento. *Rivista di Psicoanalisi* 4, 905–921.

Ferruta A. (2010). La Cassandra di Christa Wolf: tra veggenza, cecità, memoria del futuro. In Teroni S. (ed.) *Al femminile.* NICOMP L.E., Florence.

Ferruta A. (2018). Apriti sesamo. Il potere della parola. *Educazione sentimentale* 30, 36–44. Edizioni Franco Angeli.

Freud S. (1895). *Studies on Hysteria (1892–1895).* SE, 2.

Freud S. (1900). *The Interpretation of Dreams.* SE, 4–5.

Freud S. (1912). *Recommendations to Physicians Practising Psycho-Analysis.* SE, 12.

Freud S. (1923). *The Ego and the Id.* SE, 19.

Gaddini De Benedetti R. (in collaboration with Gaddini E.) (1970). Transitional Objects and the Process of Individuation: A Study in Three Different Social Groups. *J. Am. Acad. Child Psychiatry* 9, 347–365.

Gaddini E. (1980). Note sul problema mente-corpo. In *Scritti (1953–1985).* Raffaello Cortina Editore, Milan.

Gaddini E. (1985). La maschera e il cerchio. In *Scritti (1953–1985).* Raffaello Cortina Editore, Milan.

Jones E. (1959). *Free Associations: Memories of a Psychoanalyst.* Basic Books, New York.

Kaës R. (2008). *Un singolare plurale*. Borla, Rome.

Khan M. (1979). Enfance, solitude et folie. *Nouvelle Revue de Psychanalyse* 19.

Mancia M. (2004). *Sentire le parole. Archivi sonori della memoria implicita e musicalità nel transfert*. Bollati Boringhieri, Turin.

Molino A. (1997). A Conversation with Christopher Bollas. In Scalia J. (ed.) (2002). *The Vitality of Objects: Exploring the Work of Christopher Bollas*. Continuum, London and New York.

Morpurgo E. (1988). *Fra tempo e parola*. Franco Angeli, Milano.

Morpurgo E. (1998). *Chi racconta a chi?* Angeli, Milan.

Nissim Momigliano L. (1992). Supervisione e training psicoanalitico. In *Il cerchio magico*. Quaderni del Centro Milanese di Psicoanalisi "Cesare Musatti," 11, Milan 2008.

Nissim Momigliano L. (2001). *L'ascolto rispettoso*. Raffaello Cortina Editore, Milan.

Ogden T.H. (2009). *Rediscovering Psychoanalysis: Thinking and Dreaming, Learning and Forgetting*. Routledge, Hove.

Pagnoni, A. (2000). *Essere non. Il bilico dell'esistenza*. Franco Angeli,

Panksepp J. and Biven L. (2012). *The Archaeology of Mind: Neuroevolutionary Origins of Human Emotion*. Norton, New York.

Parsons M. (2007). Raiding the Inarticulate: The Internal Analytic Setting and Listening Beyond Countertransference. *Int. J. Psycho-Anal*. 88, 6, 1441–1456.

Petrella F. (1998). L'ascolto e l'ostacolo. In Egidi Morpurgo V. and Morpurgo E. (a cura dieds.).

La forma segreta. Angeli, Milan.

Petrella F. (2018). *L'ascolto e l'ostacolo*. Jaca Book, Milan.

Racalbuto A. (1994). *Tra il fare e il dire: l'esperienza dell'inconscio e del non verbale in psicoanalisi*. Raffaello Cortina Editore, Milan.

Ricoeur P. (2020). *Attorno alla psicoanalisi*. Italian edition, Barale F. (ed.) *Autour de la Psychanalyse*. Jaca Book, Milan.

Roussillon R. (2015). Un'introduzione al lavoro sulla simbolizzazione primaria. *Riv. Psicoanal*. 2, 477–491.

Roussillon R. (2018). Paradigmi per un'estensione della pratica psicoanalitica. In Bastianini T. and Ferruta A. (eds.) *La cura psicoanalitica contemporanea. Estensioni della pratica clinica*. Fioriti, Rome.

Schore A. N.(1994). *Affect Regulation and the Origin of the Self. The Neurobiology of Emotional Development* 1994; Routledge, London.

Valduga P. (1977). *Cento quartine e altre storie d'amore*. Einaudi, Turin.

Wiesel E. (1958). *Night*. Farrar, Straus, Giroux, New York, 2013.

Winnicott D.W. (1965). The Value of the Therapeutic Consultation. In Winnicott C., Shepherd R., and Davis M. (eds.) *Psycho-Analytic Explorations*. Harvard University Press, Cambridge MA, 1989.

Winnicott D.W. (1966). On the Split-off Male and Female Elements. In In Winnicott C., Shepherd R. and Davis M. (eds.) *Psycho-Analytic Explorations*. Harvard University Press, Cambridge MA, 1989.

Winnicott D.W. (1968). Unpublished correspondence with R. Gaddini.

Wolf C. (1983). *Cassandra*. Edizioni e/o, Rome 1984.

Afterword

On some aspects of contemporary psychoanalysis: beyond interpretation?

Francesco Barale

This book is about some important changes taking place in contemporary psychoanalysis.

In fact a great upheaval is happening. It is a complex phenomenon, partly "imposed" by the new clinical areas with which psychoanalysis is dealing (pathologies of identity, psychoses, borderline disturbances, autism, antisocial disturbances …), partly by historical changes and changes in contemporary forms of subjectivity itself.

Bastianini and Ferruta have already orchestrated a rich description of this in their jointly edited volume, *La cura psicoanalitica contemporanea. Estensioni della pratica clinica* (Bastianini and Ferruta 2018). Together with Guerrini Degl'Innocenti, in this new book, *Extending the Paradigm of Psychoanalytic Listening: Listening with all the Senses*, they go much further into these topics, offering a thorough reflection on how the "analysing device" can/should be rethought in the new contexts.

Just an introductory note: in this book, as in its predecessor, the word most often used to define the proposed changes (and which appears in both titles) is "extension." "Extension" suggests continuity; it indicates that those changes are happening inside the "cat's cradle" of psychoanalytic thought, that they express potentialities only partially explored, traces not developed.[1]

The allusion to the psychoanalytic *koinē* is pleasing; in certain respects it also corresponds to what is happening. Besides, the authors are careful to avoid any dichotomous thinking, making it clear that the "new" they are proposing is not "another psychoanalysis" and has not broken its bridges (epistemological and clinical) with the "old," but is work on the unresolved margins that the tradition has left us. As is well known, the question of "continuity/discontinuity" is itself the site of a traditional epistemological debate. Making clear the continuities in the apparent discontinuities of a sequence of phenomena or, vice versa, the discontinuities in the apparent continuities, depends on many things: vertices, intentions, endorsing features, magnifying lenses … (Pomian 1977). But, immediately setting these complicated questions aside as a reflective strategy in this afterword, even though they have some significance in psychopathology and in psychoanalysis too (for these, see the introductory section of Barale and Ucelli 1989), I will try to emphasise

DOI: 10.4324/9781003544647-4

above all the differences between the traditional paradigms and the mutations that are coming into being. In any case, thinking about the differences brings both the changes and the invariants into sharper focus; and in this moment of transition it is helpful to highlight what is happening, whether it be shared or not. So I will try to sketch out a first repertoire of differences.

Transference

I shall begin with one of the most "canonical" notions, which at the same time is one of those most at risk of dissolution in some recent developments. Is the notion of transference still central?

I would answer, "*Yes, but ...*" Indeed, here we have a first important "change-extension" on which the essays of all three authors shed light. In at least two directions:

First "extension"

The "traditional" transference concerns the already established representations (oedipal or pre-oedipal, pre-conscious, or repressed as the case may be) which, together with their related affects, move from the primary objects to the analyst. That repetition is classically the engine of the cure: it enables the network of meanings that have woven the histories of the subjects to be untangled, reopened, and seen anew ("*no enemy can be defeated in effigy*").

Obviously, transferential repetition has not ceased to exist. But its "material" has been markedly extended. The "new clinical practices" have provided evidence that many other things seek transformation in and through the transference: not only the repressed, the "previously established" representational dimension, *but its failures, lacunae, margins, gaps*. Whatever the nature, status, and origin of this "remainder" may be, that which is involved in the transference is, to use a Freudian term, the entire "*psychic material*," the totality of the "*unappropriated*" which the very process of symbolisation not only leaves inevitably in its wake, but actually *generates* as it occurs. This is the case *even* in the first psychic inscriptions, still undifferentiated in terms of subject–object: the pre- or proto-representational *raw material of the Id*, only very partially organised and then endlessly reorganised by secondary symbolisation.

Admittedly, this does not only happen in the "new clinical practices" or in the area of the "traumatic!" (So well illustrated in the clinical pages of this book) It is simply that the "new" practices have noisily forced us to deal with such areas, since these are where they are hyperbolically present. But this magmatic stratum of the primary process and of life is always present and always exceeds the endless attempt by representation and speech to configure it, make sense of it, give it a narrative.

If we want to address the question of *history* ("transference" and "history" are connected notions), it is not only the subject's "history" that is summoned and re-actualised in the transference, or even the multiple, more weakly expressed "micro-histories" left between the lines of the dominant history. From inside or outside or from the margins of history and micro-histories (already organised into representations) the subject's *prehistory* is also foregrounded in the transference. Green wrote that much of analytic work takes place not in the subject's "history" but in their "prehistory," in the fabric of the canvas and screen which give form and narrative to what has never entered into that "history": their "unthought future."

Can we still use the notion of "transference" for these dimensions of repetition? Yes, of course, if we want to. Transference and repetition remain fundamental phenomena, as I have said: but we should be aware that we are expanding the notion and, above all, that this "extension" of the "material" of the transference has enormous implications. Indeed, in itself it already directs the analytic situation beyond the task of revealing meanings (which have, to some extent, not yet been established). A typical notion that arises in this context is "*transformative transference*"; "transformative" not only in the sense of transforming the internal relationships with the previously established representational networks but *also* in the sense of welcoming, affective working, transition between minds, first access to the mental, first "trans-lation" (from the Latin *transferre*, which like *übersetzen*, literally means "transport," "carry beyond," i.e. transfer ...) of the mute traces of what has not yet become mental, of the "stories never told" (Ricoeur 1986).

Second extension

The "transference" is not just a transference of contents. It makes no difference whether these are presented in representational or pre-representational form, or even as *Agieren* (to which Guerrini Degl'Innocenti pays particular attention); it makes no difference whether they are already "mental" or, as I said a moment ago, still formless emotional material: even before these "contents" (whether as representations or as pre-representations), what irrupts into the transference *and is repeated* is first of all *the history of the subject's relationship with the symbolising function*, its detours, its stalemates, the attempt to reanimate the trace of an "*object for symbolising*" which allows *the symbolising apparatus* to be set in motion. Much of what happens in analysis is *a search for symbolisation and the lost object for symbolising. This, even before its contents, is the first object of the transference*. In this respect, the clinical cases cited by Bastianini, Ferruta, and Guerrini Degl'Innocenti are exemplary.

In Bionian terminology we could say that, even before single thoughts (but, I repeat, also before single proto-thoughts or single emotional turbulences) the transference is about re-vivifying the very apparatus for thinking thoughts. However, the terminology that is used ("symbolising function," "object for symbolising" ...) contains a particular stamp of the "object" that will be clarified.

As we shall see, setting nuances aside, this "extension" has further consequences for how we understand the analytic situation as a whole: it directly involves the quality of the analyst's presence as an element that may vivify – or instead replicate the failures of – the *psychic humus*, as Benedetta Guerrini calls it, which allows transformative processes to be resumed.

Associativity and listening

Following this line of thought, the "extension" of the transference brings with it an equally radical "extension-change": nothing less than a change in the "foundation stone" of the "method," the *fundamental rule*" (free-floating attention and free association).

The question is at the centre of this book, starting with the title, *Listening with all the Senses: Extending the Paradigm of Psychoanalytic Listening*, and all the authors devote intense pages to it. However, it is a delicate matter: illustrious colleagues have also reminded us recently that many things can change in psychoanalysis but, of course, "there can be no psychoanalysis without the psychoanalytic method" (Riolo 2018).

So, does this "foundation stone" still exist? "*Yes of course, but ...*" Like the transference, this fundamental feature is still there: indeed, if anything, it has been endorsed even more strongly. But within this continuity, the authors again show us some important "extensions" which undoubtedly reveal problems.

You will recall the classical schema: the fundamental rule is a particular "*epochē*" of the schemata used by the intellect in search of a mental condition that would finally be analogous to that of dream: one that should enable the network of representation underlying the phenomenological plane of consciousness to emerge.

In this case too, the classical conception was based on the idea that the *previously established* network of representations (conscious or unconscious) might guarantee that analytic work had sufficient associativity.

Let us take Freud's very famous explanation of the "fundamental rule":

> Act as though, for instance, you [the patient] were a traveller sitting next to the window of a railway carriage and describing to someone [the analyst] inside the carriage the changing views which you see outside. Finally, never forget that you have promised to be absolutely honest, and never leave anything out because, for some reason or other, it is unpleasant to tell it ...
>
> (Freud 1913, p. 135)

The genius of Freud has given us a wonderful metaphor! But think how much is already implicitly required by that situation: in the first place, that the train is moving (the instinctual impulse that sets psychic functioning in motion); and then, that the first traveller is prepared to share the consequences of this movement with the second; but even once these conditions are in place, it is necessary for the first traveller to make what is *already a double translation* of that impulse: first in visual terms (representations of something) and then as a verbal account (representation in words); and then it is necessary for the second traveller in turn to *retranslate* that account ...

To sum up: in its traditional configuration, the "fundamental rule" requires at least "a double transference onto language" (Green 1990). In fact, I would say a "triple translational transference" if we consider that even the first movement, the one that leads to visual images and the representation of something, is already a "translational" movement, and if we then restore this term to its full depth, not trivialising it as a simple transfer from one previously established semiotic code to another (Barale 2020, 2021).

But things rarely work out like this: the authors present many situations in which motor activity has not *already* been translated into representations and images; and these have not *already* been translated into language ...

As I said, on the margins of the representational network there is in fact a psyche that slips its chains, is impelled towards sense and, in order for this to happen, requires the subject of this book: an extension of the ways of listening.

This is evident to us in the example of children: nobody would ask a child to lie down on the couch and freely associate. Melanie Klein and Anna Freud showed that child analysis was possible, creating a device suited to the conditions in which children symbolise.

But as our authors illustrate, many conditions other than those of childhood (and also aspects of traditional practice with adults) impose "extensions" of listening to include other modes of expression: preverbal, musical, poetic, rhythmic, bodily ... "acts" ... the whole world of still unorganised sensoriality ...

In this case too, the authors' sophisticated knowledge of how psychoanalysis has developed as a whole avoids any simple categorising, such as "Bion versus Freud." The phenomena of traditional practice (and the constructs devised for thinking about it) have not lost their validity as a result of these "extensions," in the same way as quantum physics does not invalidate Ohm's law or classical mechanics, both of which are still indispensable for constructing a light-switch or a bridge. But most of the time, clinical work with adults is faced with polymorphous psychic amalgams: "repressed" elements of traditionally conflictual scenarios are mixed in with actions, bodily sensations, "raw" experiences of an "affective material still without a subject and object," all of which is to be "dramatised," which requires a largely pre-interpretative transformation so that a "meaning space" (Bastianini and Ferruta 2018) can be established.

Quite a few questions arise, which are the living substance of this book: how do we take all this into account and at the same time ensure that listening remains "psychoanalytic"?

Here it is enough simply to hint at the "sonic-musical" dimension which is fundamental in the very setting up of intersubjectivity, but for complex reasons (Barale and Minazzi 2008) remains extraneous to the idea of the psychic apparatus that has been handed down to us.

What is certain is the indispensability of a "polyphonic listening" that corresponds to the various levels of associativity.

This "polyphonic listening," which the authors show us at work in important examples, is certainly not "against" words and speech; it may even *enable* the word itself to "escape the prison of formal discourse" (Ferruta 2013), renewing contact with its own primal, vital, poetic, bodily, and musical matrices.

... years passed before I learned to distinguish between jumping on Papà's and Mamma's high bed, and laughter and words ...

(Meneghello 1963, p. 7)

So, it is a listening capable of reopening (in speech and in silence) the dimension that is simultaneously inside language but also before and beyond it, so that the word, as it "translates" (which is its task ...) may in turn move *towards being translated by what it translates*, and in the field of poetic speech we hear the living sound of the "voice" of the thing in question, the "constant conjunction" (as Bion called it) between pathos and logos. "[My hand] remember before
    sealing the rhyme, / you are talking about someone / who was alive and true" (Caproni 1950–1958).[2]

The device and the setting

The "extension" evoked by this "polyphonic listening" inevitably leads us to the topic of the setting, including its material features. It is one of the most sensitive topics, since this is perhaps the most clamorous point of divergence between the psychoanalytic societies (who with good reason tend to reserve the term "psychoanalysis" for the couch–chair setup and a certain minimum number of sessions each week) and a broad field of practice that has widened this definition. If the purpose of Freud's inspired invention was to facilitate the symbolic appropriation of subjective experience ("*wo Es war ...*") there is now a widespread tendency to consider it, in its material aspects, as a particular case of a more general form; useful in certain conditions, unsuitable for others.

The overall picture of the changes-extensions being described calls on us to give up the claim that patients should diligently adapt themselves to the register of secondary symbolisation; this is generally accompanied by a conception of the "analysing device" that we could call "functional."

And so, the many phenomena that trump this claim and have traditionally been thought of in "negative," if not disparaging, terms (evacuation, acting, attacks on linking and/or the setting, "anti-analysis," destructive narcissism ...) can be understood not only from the viewpoint of the destructiveness or "negativity" that infuses them (obviously this does not mean ignoring or silencing these aspects if they are present) but also – *at least also* – as the patient's attempts to get by with whatever trace of a symbolising object is available to him or her ("the patient makes do with what he has available," said Meltzer et al. 1975); and so, still more importantly, *at least also* as expressions of the need and implied search for inner interlocutors other than those who point out failures ...

Quoting Roussillon (2018) for example, Ferruta reveals how this polyphonic "extension" of listening makes it possible to get in contact with "primitive forms of communication which do not consist solely in states of evacuation or motor expression, but are also attempts to get the message across to the object about the experience of the enigmatic internal state to be integrated." But the topic is also to the fore in the fine contribution of Guerrini Degl'Innocenti centred especially on the (often ill-framed) question of "acting" and the ways in which the "embodied unconscious" is not only revealed by means of it, but resumes its "movement towards language." For her part, Bastianini devotes important pages at the start of her chapter to the need for a renewed "metapsychology of listening," trying to sketch some of its outlines, bringing interdisciplinary passion to bear on the psychoanalytic topic of how meaning is constituted from its primary intersubjective and intercorporeal bases, and intersecting this with suggestions from phenomenology and so-called "embodied hermeneutics" as well as those that derive from neurophysiological research on mirroring.

Symbolisation and the "symbolising function" of the object

On the subject of "embodied hermeneutics," let's take a step back: what does it mean to say that *"the first object of the transference is 'the symbolising function' itself?"* It could sound a bit cerebral, but this is not the case. In fact *it refers directly to the most "carnal" aspect of the analytic situation: the living search within it for the trace of the "symbolising object"* of its various responses which can get symbolisation and "subjective reappropriation" moving again.

But, as I have hinted, this shift of emphasis onto the centrality of the object has important implications for the conception of the analytic situation and the analyst's role in it.

A few theoretical notes. Of course, from the start Freud pointed to the importance of the object in constructing the psychic apparatus: but the traditional conception of symbolisation nevertheless hinges on tolerance of the object's *absence*, and the mourning for it.

Classically, to symbolise means affectively investing a representation in place of the object itself. But some say (Roussillon 2018) there is a paradox in this assumption: in order to symbolise, the object must be mourned ... but to mourn the object there needs to be an affective investment of its symbolic replacement. In other words, symbolisation! There is evidently a missing link in the chain that must be brought to light: the conditions by which symbolisation is developed first *via* the object; only later (and never entirely) in its absence. For a long time there will be a symbolisation *"through"* and *"by means of"* the object.

As has been noted, it was Winnicott above all who stressed the object's presence *"inside"* the process of symbolisation. So it is an object not only *"to be"* symbolised but also *"for"* symbolising; a paradoxical presence that allows the constitution and toleration of that otherness and that absence of which it is itself the cause. Themes like the use of the object, transitionality, illusion, and the role of the "pliable medium" (Milner 1955) are now well known.

Sometimes explicitly, more often implicitly, the authors of this book direct their and our attention towards this intermediate space. They do so without going off into complicated theoretical detours (which often suffer from over-simplification) and with a predominantly theoretical-clinical discursive strategy.

But it is nevertheless a decisive matter: in the various "extensions" being described, *this centrality of the object* delineates a psychoanalytic situation where it is *the experience of the analyst-object and the use the patient makes of it* that can reactivate the integration–symbolisation–reappropriation of aspects left at the margins of the story.

The pendulum of the transformative factors is swinging decisively towards the "experiential" and away from the cognitive. Indeed, it may swing so far in this direction that it risks destabilising the balance (which in the end is the essence of psychoanalysis) between these two poles.

I think one of the merits of this book's cultivated psychoanalytic meditation is that it succeeds in maintaining this far-from-easy balance.

Factors of transformation (cure)

Inevitably a few words must be said about "factors of transformation."

The changes are visible along at least two axes, which intersect. Each change thus reopens old questions.

1. Along the first axis, in many recent developments we have witnessed what has been called the decline of "interpretation." In fact it would be more appropriate to talk about the decline in a reductive idea of interpretation understood as "unveiling" *from the outside* (i.e. by an observer-interpreter) meanings *already* existing in the psychic mode of someone being observed (the patient) which are deciphered by the interpreter as they are masked and repeated in the transference, in dreams, etc. In the light of the extensions being described, interpretation appears more and more like the "final segment" (allowing for the fact that to some extent this is what it may always have been, as we shall see) of a complex "pre-interpretative" weaving of the very conditions of thinkability: when this final "cognitive" segment becomes possible, the transformative process has already, to a certain extent, been achieved ... We have witnessed an almost complete reversal between what was once considered the "*specific*" curative factor in psychoanalysis, its engine and heart – i.e. strict interpretation of unconscious fantasy – and what were once called "*aspecific*" or "*preparatory*" factors. If, for example, we run through the chapters on interpretation in the last great treatise on "technique" to have appeared (Etchegoyen 1986) we seem to be in another geological era with all its laying down of boundaries between "true psychoanalytic interpretation" and all the "aspecific" features (support, containment, confrontation, clarification, abreaction, explanation ...) itemised in detail; or rather, tolerated (grudgingly) as inevitable (together with the benignly non-judgemental stance) when setting up the analytical situation: but in any case merely "preparatory." Bastianini, Guerrini Degl'Innocenti, and Ferruta instead describe for us how, to a large extent, it is actually "inside" that "preliminary" dimension (before also issuing forth as "interpretation" in the classical sense) that the passage between minds takes place, a process to be

conceived of as an *aesthetic–translational–transformative–interpretative continuum*. It rests on identificatory-aesthetic bases in the analysts themselves and for a long time it is a pre-symbolic flow of attuning, sharing, *working on* the affective material – sequences of micro-variations and micro-expansions, restarts, tonal modulations – and on the harmonic-affective overall environment of cells of meaning that are being elaborated. It is also a process that may go on for a very long time, for the whole "reverberation time" (as Guerrini calls it, quoting Birksted-Breen 2005) needed so that an alphabetisation may become possible.

> Prematurely implementing an interpretation with patients who have experienced obstructive primary objects, communicating a reverie to a patient who has not yet developed sufficient alpha function, giving a metaphor to a patient who is not capable of producing their own, may carry the risk of transforming an *inter-psychic exchange* into a *trans-psychic intrusion* (Bolognini 2010) and once more occluding the natural human *drive to represent*.
>
> (Guerrini 2017)

2. Along the second axis we have witnessed the recognition of the inevitably "poietic" nature of analytic work; the decline, therefore, of that paradigm which, from 1903 (*Freud's Psycho-Analytic Procedure*, SE. 7), defined the analytic procedure solely "*per via di levare*" and never by "*porre*." The analyst-scientist dismantles defensive constructions in order to reveal the underlying psychic forces (the "taking away" of sculpture) without superimposing his own ideas onto them (the "putting on" of painting). It was the myth (albeit a benevolent one) of the analyst's "neutrality": the analytic "attitude continues to be disinterested … without exercising any influence [on the analysand] other than that of knowledge" (Etchegoyen 1986, § 25.6). The contemporary "extensions" that this book illustrates (psychoanalysis is to a great extent not only "recognition" of sense but its "constitution"; it presupposes a transition between minds which engages the analyst as a whole person) are objectively far from those canonical assumptions. Personally, as I will try to indicate, I think the evolutions represented in this book, just as they do not dispense with the question of interpretation but prompt a more complex idea of it, so they do not dispense with the dialectic between *levare* and *porre*, but call on us to think about it differently. The simple obliteration of this dialectic would expose the discipline to an objective risk of dissolving the analytic stance. And indeed a number of pages in this book testify to the striving to preserve, within a new "metapsychology of listening," the "good part" of that old dichotomy, even though it is no longer acceptable in its original formulations: see for example the beautiful pages by Ferruta "in praise of silence" which, by refraining from any excess of "interactive" intrusion, allows a truer word to appear. To be honest, I have some doubts about whether "in the old days" things really were as they are sometimes rather schematically presented (though not in this book). As far as interpretation is concerned, for example, there were already the foreshadowings of a different idea in Freud. Just

think of the whole polemic against wild interpretations (Freud 1910). Do you recall the famous joke about the uselessness of interpretations given abstractly "from outside" having "as much influence on the symptoms of nervous illness as a distribution of menu-cards in a time of famine has upon hunger" (Freud 1910, p. 225). Or the notion of *Durcharbeiten*, the long "working-through" that is needed to bring unconscious materials towards the pre-conscious and only then make them interpretable? That "almost material and intercorporeal" character of analytic *Deutung*, an inextricable interweaving of sense and force, a complex working-out of forces, affects, investments was certainly what differentiated that kind of interpretation from hermeneutics or any simple phenomenological shift of attention to the co-intentioned (Barale 2020; Ricoeur 2020). Moreover, throughout the twentieth century voices could be heard (Winnicott, Greenson, Rycroft, Klauber … it would be a long list) reminding us of something that should be quite obvious: that in the end no interpretation is effective because of its abstract "truth"; that it is attitude and affective working-through that make the comprehension of that "truth" possible … Or those who revived the importance of the analyst as a "person" (Nacht) and their "diatrophic" function (Gitelson) … Or who pointed out the need, especially when dealing with the mind's traumatic or asymbolic areas, for the concrete experience of a "new" object that might give a "different answer" (Ferenczi, Balint, Anzieu …). L. Nissim's (1985) provocation comes irresistibly to mind: "But was Freud really a Freudian?" In other words, the "cat's cradle" of psychoanalytic culture has supported and enabled multiple symbolic and intellectual games; it does not lend itself to over-simplification. If we think about it, even the most "canonical" formulations end up acknowledging the "missing link." Let's take as an example the most "canonical" canon there has ever been, one that dominated for at least half a century: Strachey's (1934) "mutative interpretations." If you have the patience to go and reread Strachey's paper you find that at the end Strachey himself wonders (I am paraphrasing), "OK, that's fine, but in the end why should 'complete' interpretations (those that astutely reconnect the transference with the internal world, the *hic et nunc* with the historical) turn out to be 'mutative'?" In fact, they too, even when sanctified by the highest authorities, may function like Freud's "menu-cards" (as indeed they often do). And his answer is: they become mutative if, by being repeated *in the relationship with the analyst*, they allow the long *introjection* of a Superego with different, more benign, qualities (NB: benign, but nevertheless still in contact with *that* internal world; the *veritative* aspect is by no means exclusive but implicit, and it remains fundamental if that sensation of benign "recognition" is to be firmly established); and so it is something intrinsically "*experiential*." Or rather, it is the inextricable mixture we will be talking about!

Intrapsychic and interpsychic

All three authors emphasise the "potentially alienating" effect, the alienating repetition, even "intrusion" (as in the quotation from Bolognini 2010) of "interpretations" that are instead given from outside and do not arise from an initial "shared experience," whose transformative path is not an expression of it. Guerrini recalls how the "inter-corporeal" dimension in which the unconscious has its roots (and which is so present throughout this book) itself highlights the uselessness of "interpreting" in that way.

The evolution that is being considered is essentially a move towards conceiving of interpretation in a less reductive way, locating it in an *aesthetic–transformative–translational–interpretative continuum* which takes its origin, strength, and substance from the levels of participation and "aesthetic" experience that the authors describe.

But if analysis is mostly not a recognition *from outside* of hidden, pre-existing meanings but "work to transform affective material" (Busacchi and Martini 2020), a third axis of changes comes into view: *where and how does this transformation happen?*

Here we must address (and discuss …) other evolutions which we only have time to name.

First, the gradually extended function of the "countertransference": from Heimann and Racker, passing through the contributions of so many other important writers (among whom I will only recall Nissim in Milan, and for reasons that are personal more than scientific) to an idea of countertransference that little by little becomes not only a place for recognition but for "metabolising" what the analyst receives …

And then later evolutions: the idea of the "field" as the site of a transformation that comes neither from the analyst's external knowledge nor from a simple rein-trojection of something appearing in the countertransference, but something that *happens* in a trans-personal dimension.

And along the same lines, interest in the "analytic third" (Ogden 2009); or the "interpsychic" to which Bolognini (2008) has devoted wonderful analyses …

Finally, the rooting of these changes in post-Bionian perspectives, which have found some of their most notable and significant expressions here in Italy (Ferro and Civitarese 2015; Civitarese and Ferro 2020).

But although we cannot follow all these developments now, their traces are spread throughout this text in their most fertile forms.

Problems and questions

Moving away from the book by Bastianini, Ferruta, and Guerrini, I will confine myself to pointing out some new fronts opened up by the evolutions they describe.

My starting point is the best-known model: the post-Bionian idea of analysis as a "field," a transpersonal, dreaming situation which transforms beta elements into alpha, expands the apparatus for thinking thoughts, and creates ("co-constructs") the unconscious before revealing it…

This important model is still in a happy state of expansion. Which in itself prompts a reflection on its problematic margins.

Without going into a discussion of its basic assumptions, the first problem that arises is: *how does the "return journey" work?*

Which is to say: when that transpersonal situation has transformed material into dream, how does it come to form part of *the subject's specific heritage,* of their *personal* subjective experience? When all is said and done, from that kaleidoscopic and contrapuntal interweaving of elements with various origins which has taken shape "in the field," which part of what specifically concerns the subject – their internal reality, their Self, memory, history, *bios* – will be laid down lastingly in their internal world, and how? *How do we return to the intrapsychic?*

The point is not as banal as it may seem. It prompts complicated theoretical questions which I won't tackle now (to give just a few examples: the "group" structure of the Self, whose radical otherness we have always inhabited; the hypothesis of a "metapsychology of the third type"; the great theme of the "traces" of the internal history ... etc.). Significant contributions have recently appeared on this subject, from a variety of vertices and perspectives (Bolognini 2019; Rossi and Ruggiero 2018).

In any case, it seems insufficient to reply that the "introjection" of the "dreaming" mental functioning that has been experienced and of what has been transformed (or rather, "created") in the transpersonal "field" will simply happen. In fact, what is in question are the conditions, modes, and function of this "re-appropriation," in its dialectic with the system of "traces" around which the narrative of the internal story is organised.

If we head in this direction, we end up bumping into the Winnicottian notion of "subjective appropriation" founded on the transpersonal matrix, which is in fact decisive for the way we conceive the analytic situation and its function.

Patients come to us suffering from something. The basic assumption of psychoanalysis is that this suffering (for example, always getting into the same unfortunate situations ...) has to do with *what is unappropriated in their stories*. Our patients suffer (as we all do to some extent ...) from what is unappropriated in their/our stories ... This does not mean simply widening the scope of Freud's dictum that "hysterics suffer from forgetting" (i.e. the neurotic phenomenon is the expression of something repressed) to include all psychic material (based on the "extensions" considered above). We have established in the meantime that "what has not been appropriated in our history" and causes us suffering is not only the repressed but also that which has never found access, has never been thought and narrated.

From this point of view, in the words of Ricoeur cited earlier, analysis is the "possibility of reprising histories (and prehistories) that have never been told." Not in general, though: they must be *those particular histories and prehistories,* the ones of those particular patients *in all their singularity and distinctiveness*; not other ones, even if they are more satisfying.

And so some fundamental questions present themselves.

In this context, we inevitably recall Laplanche's harsh, lapidary criticism that, in the end, any "psychoanalytic narratology" risks becoming an expedient way to tame the radical "otherness" which psychoanalysis must confront; a way of "balancing the books," of introducing fictitious coherences: "psychoanalysis is by definition an anti-narrative." This admonition (which actually "overshoots the mark": Barale 2020) is nevertheless a resonant reminder of analytic work's inescapable bond with what is outside the discursive-interpretative universe (and also outside any "intersubjective field"): the dimension of the other. The other inside ourselves: the irreducible otherness, singularity, historicality, and materiality of the other that we encounter and with whom we are concerned; the other who, from outside and inside, keeps loading us up with affective material, memory, history. In Laplanche's admonition there was the idea that the psychoanalytic process must reject an autarkic notion of the discursive universe and avoid any swerve in the direction of "creationism." The interminable remodelling of the affective material is nevertheless still an attempt to translate the traces of what is outside and prior to any intersubjective "field." Its "trails" as Corrao called them.

Laplanche's critique threw the baby out with the bathwater (Barale 2020) but was certainly justified in relation to any "narratology" which disarticulated the dialectic between "narrative truth" and "historical truth" instead of reopening and keeping open the tension in the "intermediate province" of the analytic situation; an "intermediate province" that this book shows us in all its unexpected extension and its multitude of dimensions and pathways.

So we are presented with the problem of how to keep in mind, at least suspended, a reference to the patient's reality and inner story, and a *veritative* striving towards them without "taking them over," ensuring that we maintain our "negative capability." It is part of this analytic attitude of respect for the "other." If, by contrast, these references (with all the critical aspects that we know well …), instead of remaining "in suspension," are considered irrelevant (or even an obstacle to the transformations that occur in the "interpsychic"): that is to say, if the dialectic between narrative truth and historical truth is disarticulated, the "return journey to the intrapsychic" and "subjective reappropriation" are not facilitated.

In essence, after all the transpersonal interchanges wonderfully described by some evolutions of contemporary psychoanalysis, we are again faced with the demand that, in the midst of them, we do not lose sight of the intrapsychic, the person's individuality, their history; their ipseity, and with it the radical otherness that inhabits them and us.

It is certainly not only a "theoretical" question: it stands at the living heart of "use of the analyst-analysis-object."

Still on the topic of "subjective reappropriation," another delicate point about the evolutions in progress, connected to the previous one, is represented by the current shift towards "*porre*" and the "poietic" function of analysis and analysts. Here too a well-tempered dialectic fosters a *narrative humus* in which "stories never told" can be taken up and continued. Its disarticulation can instead cause a slippage towards excessive constructionism and a fantasy of creating "new" narratives that lose their ties to a patient's specific subjectivity, their reality, the traces of their history, their *bios*. Paradoxically, and despite the best intentions, this can replicate the effects of the "occupation" by the primary objects.

Among the many fronts opened up by the evolutions of contemporary psychoanalysis which this wonderful book has told us about, it is worth recalling just one more (since I should be coming to a close), connected to the idea of the analyst as a "new object." It is an aspect that emerged recently in a work by De Masi (2021) on analyses that tend to get more and more prolonged. Why does this happen? Because pathologies are more complicated? *Yes, maybe this too*. But in the first place, isn't it the aims and expectations of analysis that are changing?

The "end" of analysis as its *goal* and the "end" as its *termination* are closely connected. If the aim of analysis becomes the reanimation of deficient or absent mental presences and functions and the analyst's aim becomes that of offering themselves as a new "transformative" (if not "replacement") object, this inevitably raises the risk of encouraging feelings of "grandiosity" in the analyst, major idealisation, indispensability.

It's an almost inevitable risk, within certain limits, in the evolutions that we have described, but for this very reason we must be fully aware of it, if only to moderate it from the outset.

Essentially, we are at a watershed moment in the old question of corrective experience; the analyst's involvement in the analytic process becomes highly sensitive and imposes great, indeed countertransferential, responsibilities.

So the sea of contemporary psychoanalysis is rich in fascinating evolutions through which this book magisterially guides us; but also full of sandbanks and perils.

Fortunately, there are guidelines to help us navigate.

First of all, the image of the Winnicottian mother (with, oh dear yes, all the caveats! …) who is not only capable of attunement, acceptance, restoration, and of functioning as a "pliable medium" for the transitional area… but does all this while maintaining the child's sensation that *they themselves* are finding/creating their own reality: who steps back as soon as she can and does not impose herself on this "*invention*"… and who, in the most profound attunement, also moves towards separateness and triangulation, being equipped, one hopes, with an "oedipal function of the mind" (Di Chiara 1985).

Corresponding to this is the image of an analyst intent on avoiding any excessive constructionism or interventionism, not imposing his or her creative imagination or reverie (or that of the "field") on the patient's world … Ready not only to share, to facilitate a dreaming climate, but also to withdraw into the background, as soon as he or she has fulfilled the function of supporting the patient's "subjective reappropriation." In the end it is what Winnicott (1971, p. 85) meant by his famous admission, "It appals me to think how much deep change I have prevented or delayed in patients *in a certain classification category* by my personal need to interpret."

Di Chiara (2024) describes the encounter between the analyst's "internal psychoanalytic narrator" and the "internal narrator" of the patient, which is often still rudimentary and overwhelmed by the untranslatable. This encounter is set up by sharing very primitive levels of identification and aesthetic "feeling." Then a mutual exchange gradually develops, sustained by the analyst's ability to nurture and support the patient's nascent narrative without ever imposing themselves on it but using the "provisional constructions" of their own narrative, ready to withdraw them, maintaining a "constant conjunction" between pathos and logos, holding and thinking, between the unrepresentable and a striving towards sense, and between deep sharing and respectful acknowledgement of the other's irreducible otherness; between experience and knowledge.

Finally, it was Klauber who, 50 years ago in *Difficulties in the Analytic Encounter* (Klauber 1981), called the analyst a "reanimator of Eros" in the patient's world. Eros obviously has the capacity for linking, affective investment, sense … without getting scared if all this also makes its way into the scenes of transference and countertransference; but taking care "always to withdraw into the background" of the scene as soon as possible, and not occupying the "field." This is a really difficult mixture of capacity, profound presence, and "*exiting the scene*:" but it is yet another fundamental mixture in the strange art of psychoanalysis …!

What is there "beyond interpretation?" I would say: there is a slightly more complex idea of the multiple dimensions and conditions of the *aesthetic–transformative–translational–interpretative continuum*, towards sense and narrative, and of that "to be translated" (Laplanche 1998) that is the unconscious (and as are our own lives).

Serra del Monte, August 2021

Notes

1 The metaphor of the game of the "cat's cradle" was coined by E. Gombrich in 1971 in relation to the development of artistic forms and languages. "There is an element in all art – and certainly in all Western art – which might for brevity's sake be called the 'cat's cradle' element. Art … is born of art. The young artist takes over the game from his predecessors and as he does so he introduces variations. In Western communities, at least, art has thus become a social game played among the artists and the pattern that emerges with each move owes at least as much to the moves that have gone before as it owes to the ingenious variation introduced by the present player." In psychoanalysis the metaphor was taken up by Neri 1979 for the mental activity of the group; recently also by Barale 2021, in its dialectic with negative capability.)

2 Mia mano, fatti piuma:
fatti vela; e leggera
muovendoti sulla tastiera,
sii cauta. E bada, prima
di fermare la rima,
che stai scrivendo d'una
che fu viva e fu vera. (Caproni 1950–1958)

References

Barale F. (2020). Introduzione a P. Ricoeur (1954–2003) *Attorno alla psicoanalisi*. Jaca Books, Milan 2020.

Barale F. (2021a). Pàthei Màthos. Prima della narrazione e oltre: fragilità umana, tragico e psicoanalisi in 3 scritti "minori" di P. Ricoeur, tra la "piccola etica" e l'oblio. *Babel*, October 2021.

Barale F. and Minazzi V. (2008). Off the Beaten Track: Freud, Sound and Music. Statement of a Problem and Some Historico-Critical Notes. *Int. J. Psycho-Anal.* 89, 937–957.

Barale F. and Ucelli di Nemi S. (1989). Il vaso di Pandora. Riflessioni sull'esperienza psicotica acuta. In De Martis D. (ed.) *La crisi psicotica acuta*. Borla, Rome.

Bastianini T. and Ferruta A. (eds.) (2018). *La cura Psicoanalitica contemporanea. Estensioni della pratica clinica*. Fioriti, Rome.

Birksted-Breen D. (2005). The feminine. In *Introducing Psychoanalysis*. Routledge, London, 142–152

Bolognini S. (2008). *Secret Passages: The Theory and Technique of Interpsychic Relations*. Hove, Routledge, 2011.

Bolognini S. (2019). *Vital Flows Between the Self and Non-Self: the Interpsychic*. Routledge, Abingdon, 2022.

Busacchi V. and Martini G. (2020). *L'identità in questione. Saggio di psicoanalisi e ermeneutica*. Jaca Book, Milan.

Caproni G. (1950–1958). Il seme del piangere. In *Tutte le poesie*. Garzanti, Milan 1990.

Civitarese G. and Ferro A. (2020). *Vitalità e gioco in psicoanalisi*. Cortina, Milan.

Corrao F. (1998). *Orme*. Cortina, Milan.

De Masi F. (2021). *Le analisi che si prolungano*. Paper presented at the Centro Milanese di Psicoanalisi, February 2021.

Di Chiara G. (1985). Una prospettiva del dopo Freud: un posto per l'altro. *Riv. Psicoan*. 29, 451–461.

Di Chiara G. (2024). *Il dono dell'altro. Origine, funzioni e destino del narratore psicoanalitico*. Jaca Book, Milan.

Etchegoyen R.H. (1986). *The Fundamentals of Psychoanalytic Technique*. Routledge, Abingdon 2018.

Ferro A. and Civitarese G. (2015). *Il campo analitico e le sue trasformazioni*. Cortina, Milan.

Freud S. (1903). *Freud's Psycho-analytic Procedure*. SE. 7.

Freud S. (1910). *"Wild" Psycho-analysis*. SE. 11.

Freud S. (1913). *On Beginning the Treatment: Further Recommendations on the Technique of Psychoanalysis I*, SE. 12.

Gombrich E. (1971). Freud's Aesthetics. In Kurzweil E. and Philips S.W. (eds.) *Literature and Psychoanalysis*. Columbia University Press, New York, 1983.

Green A. (1990). *Psicoanalisi degli stati limite. La follia privata*. Cortina, Milan 1991.

Guerrini degl'Innocenti B. (2017). Rappresentazione in azione. Stati non rappresentati della mente e trasformazione simbolica. *Riv. Psicoan*. 63, 3, 573–590.

Klauber J. (1981). *Difficulties in the Analytic Encounter*. Routledge, Abingdon 2018.

Laplanche J. (1998) Narratività e ermeneutica. *Ricerca psicoanalitica* XI, 1, 7, 2000.

Meneghello L. (1963). *Libera nos a Malo*. Feltrinelli, Milan.

Meltzer D., Bremner J., Hoxter S., Weddell D. and Wittenberg I. (1975). *Explorations in Autism: A Psycho-Analytical Study*. Harris Meltzer Trust.

Milner M. (1955). The role of illusion in symbol formation, in *The Suppressed Madness of Sane Men*. Routledge, Abingdon 1987.

Nissim L. (1985). Una stagione a Vienna: ma Freud era freudiano? In Robutti A. (ed.) *L'ascolto rispettoso. Scritti psicoanalitici*. Cortina, Milan 2001.

Neri C. (1979). Rappresentazione, costruzione, interpretazione nel gruppo. *Gruppo e funzione analitica* I, 1, 31–51.

Pomian K. (1977). Entry on Catastrophes. In *Enciclopedia Einaudi*. Einaudi, Turin.

Ricoeur P. (1986). La vita. Un racconto in cerca di un narratore. In Barale F. (ed.) *Attorno alla psicoanalisi*. Jaca Book, Milan 2020.

Ricoeur P. (2020). Attorno alla psicoanalisi. In F. Barale (ed.) *Attorno alla psicoanalisi*. Jaca Book, Milan 2020.

Riolo F. (2018). Il metodo psicoanalitico e i suoi funtori. In Bastianini T. and Ferruta A. (eds.) *La cura Psicoanalitica contemporanea. Estensioni della pratica clinica*. Fioriti, Rome.

Rossi N, Ruggiero I. (2018). *Transpsichico, interpsichico, intrapsichico*. Teoria e clinica. F. Angeli, Milan.

Roussillon R. (2018). Paradigmi per un'estensione della pratica psicoanalitica. In Bastianini T. and Ferruta A. (eds.) *La cura psicoanalitica contemporanea*. Fioriti, Rome.

Strachey J. (1934). The Nature of the Therapeutic Action of Psycho-Analysis. *Int. J. Psychoanal.* 15, 127–159.

Winnicott D.W. (1971). *Playing and Reality*. Tavistock, London.

Index

absence, dissimulation 35
absolute analytic listening 74–75
absolute listening 71–73
acting-out 12; analyst discussions 19
action 49; agent (plural subject) 60;
    beginning 47, 57–59; being in action
    53; metapsychology 19; pattern,
    extrapolation 54; pre-representation/
    proto-representation 58; psychic action,
    configuration 18; representations 55–56;
    representations in action 53; shift 56–57;
    specific form 17–18; theory, absence 19
adverse experiences, impact 29
aesthetic-transformative-translational-
    interpretative continuum 113, 117
aesthetic-translational-transformative-
    interpretative continuum 111
affective auto-regulation/hetero-
    regulation, forms construction 11
affective communication: occurrence 14;
    urgency 27
affective investment: intensities, listening
    1; qualities/quantities 2–3
affective material 111
affective orders, compatibility relations 12
affective overflow, feeling 48
affective record, shared repetition
    in action 32
affective registration, forms 29
affective state: incorporation 34;
    perception, motoric accompaniment 22
affective status, incorporation 34
affective symbolisation 31
affectivity, display 54–55
affect, quantity 5
African American slaves, blues
    singing 39

aggressiveness, externalisation 17
Agieren concept 24
alphabetisation, possibility 111
alphabet, presence 3
alpha elements: formation 113;
    proliferation 65
alpha function 111
Alvarez, Anne 78, 84
a-modal symbolic mental representations,
    activation 60
analysing device: conception/setting
    108–109; rethinking 103
analysing function 48
analysis: post-Bionian idea 113; word,
    importance 86
Analysis Terminable and Interminable
    (Freud) 30–31
analyst(s): dangers, patient repressed
    material (impact) 31; decentring
    75; enchanting/hypnotising 34;
    internal psychoanalytic narrator,
    encounter 116–117; mental position,
    discussion 88–89; mental processes,
    metapsychology 5; neutrality 111; new
    object, equivalence 116; object-subject
    presence 76; psyche-soma 31; psychic
    movement, creation 9; receiving,
    metabolising 113; relationship 112;
    symbolising listening 38
analyst-analysis object, usage 115
analyst-object: experience 110; physical
    presence, impact 75
analyst-patient, dialogue (occurrence) 80
analytic *Deutung,* material/intercórporeal
    character 112
analytic device 55–56
analytic dialogue, openness 89

analytic listening 69–70, 72; condition, paradox 77; function 8–9; openness 75; quality, investigations 70; usage 16
analytic probes, enquiry 4
analytic relationship 49; offering 71; "work as a double" 21
analytic set-up 2
analytic space, transferential reawakenings (invasion) 16–17
analytic third, interest 113
analytic work, poietic nature (recognition) 111–112
anger, revelation 33
annihilation, feeling (pervasiveness) 36
anorexia, tendencies 62
anti-analysis 108
Antigone, Polyneices (blood-tie) 92
anti-narrative 114–116
anxiety: defence 33, 52; generation 18; translation 16
Anzieu, Didier 77, 93–96
appropriation, involvement 11
"aspecific" features, boundaries 110
associative modes, usage 77–78
associative psychic work 39
associative thought, concept 10
associativity: listening, relationship 106–108; plural forms 13–14
assonances, echo (reliance) 50–51
asymmetry, appearance 94
attention: analyst focus 76; directing 59; intentional attention 72; suspended attention 72
attitude, changes 21
auditory dimension, privilege 73–74
Aulagnier, Piera 77
author, character search 56, 65
auto-regulation, forms construction 11
avoidance: defence 78; processes 69–70

Babighian, Gregorio 89–90
background noise 55
"balancing the books" 114–115
becoming, formulation 9
behavioural phenomena 60
being in action 53
being in relation, narrative form 58
being in things 54
being-not 74
Benedetto, Antonio di 84
benign curiosity 75
benign recognition, sensation 112

beta elements, transformation 113
bios, traces 115
blockages, creation 76–77
Blue in Green (Davis) 37–38
blue note: listening 36–40; musical sign 37–38
blues singing 39
bodily Self, founding nucleus 57–58
bodily surface information, elements 20
body: enigmatic/potent symptom 63; knowledge, clinical reflections 31–36; periphery, grey masses (relationship) 3; psyche, caesura 24; psychosomatic disorders 34; scheme 26; speaking 61; starvation 62; usage, sequence indications 10
body-mind (action) 57
Bogart, Humphrey 73
bond: building, reciprocity (impact) 92; faith 13; familial bonds, strength/importance 91–92; prisoner 79; sibling bond, example 90, 91–93
borderline states, clinical work 12
Borutti, Silvana 92
Boston Change Process Study Group (BCPSG) 28
boundary, creation 13
breakdown, approach 78–79
Brook, Peter 93
Brooks, Richard 73
bubble, individual (equivalence) 34

caesura: bridging 23; investigation, question 23–28; passage 24; penetration 24
cannibal subjectivity 76
caregiving, experience 55
case reports, emphasis 81
castoff 86
catastrophe, threshold 39
cat's cradle (psychoanalytic culture) 112
cerebral cortex, fibre tracts (impact) 3
change, occurrence 27
changes-extensions 108
chaos, edge 49–50
children, self-perception 33
Chodorow, Nancy 81
Chopin, Frederic 38
classification category 116
clinical care, goals 2
clinical comprehension, capacity (widening) 9

clinical practice, extension 21–22
closeness, elements 20
co-associativity 19
coexistence levels 37
coherences, introduction 114–115
comfort, providing 54
communicable derivatives 80
communication: capability 60;
    centrality 84; contents, access 31–34;
    intersubjective communication, listening
    81; linguistic communication 59;
    metaphorical sense, catching (inability)
    63; multiple codes 27–28; penetration
    24; primitive forms 108–109; psychic
    work 5; speech communication 59–61;
    symbolic/non-symbolic codes 21;
    verbal/non-verbal communication,
    usage 84
communicative play 8
communicative registers, multiplicity 4
compatibility, relations (discovery) 12
complex sounds, articulation 59
condensation: communicable derivative 80;
    mechanisms 81
condensed words, listening 80
conflict: interpersonal situations 33;
    network 30; resolving/working,
    reparative potential 13
confusion: connotations 50; defence
    characteristics 52
con-fusion, experiences (inducing) 51
connections/consonances, impact 8
conscious: post-natal conscious, direction
    24; qualities, reserving 23–24
consciousness: acts 23; attainment 21;
    dyadic expansion, hypothesis 7–8;
    individual state, extension 8; intrusion
    34; perception-consciousness,
    conceptual binomial (openness) 10–11;
    quality 26; surface 81
constant conjunction 108; maintenance 117
constant dialogue, object presence
    (quality) 29
constructionism, excess 115
"Constructions in Analysis" (Freud) 30
container (Skin-Ego function) 96
continuity/discontinuity, question 103
core relatedness domain, experience 25
correlation, process (heterogeneity) 5
counterinvestments, network 30
countertransference 48; construct 33;
    dreaming 56; extended function 113

couple object 16–17
COVID-19, reflections 36–40
cryptic messages, identification/
    decoding 81

Davis, Miles 37
Deadline (movie) 73
deafness, impact 89
death instinct 29
defence, characteristics 52
defensive dissociation 36
defensive set-ups, weakening 70
deficit, traumas 29
deictic use 59
Delacroix, Eugene 38
delirium, triggering 30
denial: defence 78; opportunity 17
denied suffering 90–91
depersonalisation 87
derivation, process (heterogeneity) 5
dermatitis, defence 94
despair, unnameable states 34
destructive narcissism 108
destructiveness, viewpoint 108
diachrony, synchrony (contrast) 71
diagnostic ability, refinement 48
dialogue: complexity, issues 28;
    intervention cessation, request 76
diatrophic function 112
Difficulties in the Analytic Encounter
    (Klauber) 117
discursive interpretation 86
discursive-interpretative universe, analytic
    work (bond) 115
displacement (communicable derivative) 80
dissemination 69–70
dissociated memory system,
    establishment 34
dissociated places 34–36
dissociation 78; strategy 33–34
distance, elements 20
disturbances, translation 16
domination: absence 72; dynamic 16
Donnet, Jean-Luc 72, 77
double translation 106, 107
dread, unnameable states 34
dream-elements 80
dreaming mental function, introjection 114
dream, seed 5
dream-thoughts, translation 80
dream-work 11, 80; model,
    word-representations 77

drive-object pairing, indivisibility 10
Dumas, Alexandre 38
Durcharbeiten 112
dyadic expansion, hypothesis 8
dynamic psychoanalysis 92

early trauma, imprint 34
economic factor, concept 14
economic-semiotic mode 5
edgedness, feeling 6
Ego (ego): derivation 6; immaturity 15;
    integration, problem 14; restriction 30;
    splitting-dissociation, states 30
Ego and the Id, The (Freud) 24
Ego-structuring, foundation (integration
    question) 13–15
"Egyptian dream book" (Freud) 47
Einfall (Freud) 56
elaboration, failure (elaboration) 34
embodied hermeneutics 109
embodied listening 2
embodied mechanisms/approach 60–61
embodied simulation, theory 61
embodied unconscious 109
embodied unconsciousness 47
embryonic emotional vitality 78
embryonic No, toleration (analyst
    capability) 17
emergent relatedness domain,
    experience 25
"emergings" 71
emotion: emergence 78; expression 27;
    frost 32
emotional communication, occurrence 14
emotional contact, desire 69
emotional histories, object encounter 22–23
emotional neglect, feeling (experience) 32
emotional schemata, transcription 33
emotional states, inexpressibility 31
emotional survival, strategy 33–34
empathy, concept 26
emptiness, phenomena 30
enactment 49, 55–56; construct 33;
    hypothesis 65; resonances 9; traumatic
    memory enactments 61
enclosed spaces, claustrophobic fear 79
encounter: hallucination 13; singular
    reverberations 22
endogenous sensory stimuli, usage 6
enemy, defeat (impossibility) 104
enigmatic privacy 88
environmental pressure, increase 34

epistemophilic instinct (Klein) 7
"*epochē*" 106
erotic dynamics 15
Essere non. Il bilico dell'esistenza
    (Being-not. Existence as balance) 74
event, memory 82
evidence (collection), senses (usage) 5
excess: listening 28–31; traumas 29
excitations, production 27
existence, continuity 29
exogenous sensory stimuli, usage 6
expansion, happy state 113
experience: beginnings 56–57; integration/
    non-integration 13–14; presentations 58;
    psychic form 56–57
experiential context, pre-emptive/injunctive
    mode 76–77
experiential potentialities, development 71
exploratory schemata, usage 73–74
*Extending the Paradigm of Psychoanalytic
    Listening: Listening with all the Senses*
    (Bastianini/Ferruta/Degl'Innocenti) 103
extension(s) 103; constitution 111;
    evocation, polyphonic listening (impact)
    108–109; first extension 104–105;
    imposition 107; second extension 105
external object: existence/aliveness/
    behaviour 13; splitting-dissociation
    characterisation 16

facial expression (usage), sequence
    indications 10
Faimberg, Haydée 70, 75–76
familial bonds, strength/importance 91–92
fantasying, stasis 15
fear, unnameable states 34
feelings: containment 21; names 21
"feeling words" 84
feet (usage), sequence indications 10
fibre tracts, impact 3
figurability, evocation 54
flesh, language 27
flight 34–36
flute/triangle, open space 93
forced interpretations 79
formless, form (giving) 55–56
"found-created," illusion (role) 29
fragmentation, connotations 50
free associations 85, 106; concept 10;
    information, supply 9; pathway 76
*Free Associations: Memories of a
    Psychoanalyst* (Jones) 80

free-floating attention 85, 106
Freud, Anna 107
Freud, Sigmund 12, 14, 106, 109, 112;
  Agieren concept, usage 24; *Analysis
  Terminable and Interminable* 30–31;
  "Constructions in Analysis" 30; death
  instinct 29; *Ego and the Id, The* 24;
  "Egyptian dream book" 47; *Einfall*
  56; events, traces 14; fundamental rule
  106; *Interpretation of Dreams, The* 6,
  80; *Interpretation of the Aphasias, The*
  3; language, impact 2; menu-cards,
  function 112; *Moses and Monotheism*
  30; *Nebenmensch* (nearest human being)
  56; *Negation* 18; "On Psychotherapy"
  40; *Outline of Psychoanalysis* 24;
  psyche (mental life), continuum
  23; *Remembering, Repeating, and
  Working-Through* 12; *Studies on
  Hysteria* 82; *Traumdeutung* 58; *Two
  Principles of Mental Functioning* 10–11;
  Verwerfung concept 34
Fubini, Mario 87
functional changes, elements (impact) 3
functioning, psychic ways 70
fundamental rule: configuration,
  requirement 106–107; Freud
  explanation 106
Fusini, Nadia 3

Gaddini, Eugenio 48, 94
Gaddini, Renata 90
Gaddini, Renata De Benedetti 94
gain, power (demonstration) 83
Galland, Antoine 83
generative enactments 19
Geography is the Remedy (Pirandello) 35
Gestalt parameters, response 73–74
gestural language 59
gestures 22–23; human usage 59
Glegerian ambiguities 85
going mad, anxiety 49
grandiosity, feelings (encouragement) 116
gratification: need 54; providing 51
Greeks, word/concept 92
Grid, The (Bion) 83

hallucinating (data functioning/gathering
  register) 5
hallucination: negative hallucination 16;
  predisposition, unification 13;
  triggering 30

handling (maternal care) 94
handling, discussion 87
hands (usage), sequence indications 10
"hearing of hearing" (knowing of
  knowing) 24
heterogenous patients, recalling 48–49
heterogenous psychic communications,
  connection 8
heterogenous psychic materials, listening
  (impact) 5
heterological constitution,
  acknowledgement (need) 92
hetero-regulation, forms construction 11
historical dimensions, psychic dimensions
  (correlation) 13
historical thickness 4
history (histories): arrival, pre-emptive/
  injunctive mode 76–77; margins 105;
  trace 6; transference, connection
  104–105
holding (maternal care) 94
homeostatic equilibrium, loss 57
Homo sapiens, phonatory apparatus
  (evolution) 59
hope, logic 13
humanity, catastrophe (threshold) 39
husband, traumatic loss 31–32
hybrid psychosomatic dimensions 77
hysterical symptoms 82, 91

iconic function, acquisition 58
iconic use 59
idealisation (defensive strategy) 52
identification, concept 26
identification/counter-identification,
  short-circuiting 53
idiom, safeguarding 36
Id, raw material 104
illusion 109; role 12
imagination, directing 59
imaginative, pre-symbolic (relationship) 22
imagining (data functioning/gathering
  register) 5
imitation, concept 26
immediacy, qualities 81–82
impasse, types 19
implicit knowing, consideration 20
implicit memory 11; neural circuits,
  discovery 33
implicit relational knowledge 11
impotence, experience 12
imprisonment, freedom 79

impulse: contradiction/conflict 37; double
    translation 106
individual: bubble, equivalence 34;
    development, integration (inability) 14
individuation (Skin-Ego function) 96
infant: pre-representational affectivity
    57; transitional object, usage
    (relationship) 13
infantile experiences, registration 33
Inferno (Dante) 87
informal art *(arte povera)* 72
information (collection), senses (usage) 5
inner speech 25
instinctual impulse, strength 21
instinctual reawakening 63
instruction, cognitive logic 86
integrated body-ego 57
integration, loss 87
intellectualised communication, impact 81
intelligibility tools 24
intentional attention 72
intentional comprehension, non-linguistic
    infrastructure 59
intentionality, acknowledgement
    (failure) 54
intentions, agent (plural subject) 60
inter-action, reduction 51
interbrain synchronisation 4
intercorporeal dimension, origins 113
intercorporeal functioning 27
intercorporeality, presence 61
interests, complementarity
    (maintenance) 91
internal analytic setting 73
internal change 27
internal/external mother, curing 79
internal inspiration, speaking (link) 86
internal narrator (patient) 116–117
internal object: dispersal in suspension 56;
    splitting-dissociation characterisation
    16; transitional object (infant usage) 13
internal object-analyst, relationship 53
interpersonal experience, simultaneous
    forms 25
interpretation: decline 110–111; object 73
Interpretation of Dreams, The (Freud) 6, 80
*Interpretation of the Aphasias,
    The* (Freud) 3
inter-psychic exchange, transformation
    risk 111
interpsychic function 27
interpsychic functioning 112–113

intersensoriality (Skin-Ego function) 96
intersubjective communication, listening 81
intersubjective construction, forms
    (listening) 20–22
intersubjective context, defining 60
intersubjective field (construct) 33
intersubjective functioning 27
intersubjective relatedness domain,
    experience 25
intersubjective resonance 2
intersubjectivity (construct) 33
into-form 54
intrapsychic functioning 27, 112–113
intrapsychic plane, experience
    (pervasiveness) 32
intrapsychic return 115
intrapsychic transformation 66
investments, network 30
island-words, sonic material 73–75
isolation: defence 78; inducing 76

joint attentional frame 60
joint psychic work 9
Jones, Ernest 80
judgement, first form 17

"kaleidoscopic room" 37
kinetics, elements 20
Klein, Melanie 107
K-link 7
knowing, type 20
knowledge: goals 2; implicit relational
    knowledge 11; *primum movens* 57;
    refinement 48; terminal points, direct
    relation 23
koinē, allusion 103
Kulturarbeit 15

*La cura psicoanalitica contemporanea.
    Estensioni della pratica clinica*
    (Bastianini and Ferruta) 103
language: bodily ingredients 25; category,
    traces (relationship) 17–18; centrality
    26; development, sacrifice 25;
    double-edge sword 25; function,
    recovery 87; impact 2; impoverishment
    62–63; link 86; location 25; movements
    109; speaking, differences 77; usage,
    risk 87
language-actions 64
L'ascolto rispettoso (Momigliano) 75
La tentazione (Temptation), poem 87–88

Le Moi-peau (The Skin-Ego) (Anzieu) 93
levare, porre (dialectic) 111–112
libidinal energy 63
life: breath 73; event, avoidance 69;
    exigencies 27; importance, attachment
    91; search, impossibility 79; senseless
    chaos 52; unconscious living 78
life-story production, plastic clarity 11
linguistic communication 59
linguistic symbolisation 14
listening: absolute listening 71–73;
    analytic listening 72; associativity,
    relationship 106–108; capacity 77;
    embodied listening 2; metapsychology,
    renewal 5; musical listening 84;
    polyphonic extension 108–109;
    position, adoption 1; quality 73;
    quasi-hallucinatory quality 77; readiness
    72; relationship imprisonment 72;
    "respectful listening" 70; senses, usage
    1; silence, connection 88–90
"listening to listening" 70
lived experience, progress 13
Lives of Others, The (movie) 90
living discourse, examination 31
"living laboratory" 37
living transferential element, listening/
    catching 79
living witnesses: flight comprehension 36;
    impact 36
loneliness: cold 97; unnameable states 34

Magic Flute, The (Brook production) 93
"magic" word, power 82–88
Mancia, Mauro 84
"Mask and the Circle, The" (Gaddini/
    Gaddini) 94
maternal care, impact 94
meaning(s): absolute listening 71–73; cells,
    harmonic-affective environment 111;
    generation 7; scrap 51
meaning cells, harmonic-affective
    environment 111
meaning space 107
means, ends (relationship) 50–51
meeting paradigm 38
memories in feelings 65
memory (memories): multiple signs, system
    17–18; primitive personal memory 36;
    recollection, absence 30
me/not-me, distinction (achievement) 56
mental attunement 59

mental capacity, lengthening 72
mental function, introjection 114
mental impression 54
mental life, knowledge 23
menu-cards, function (Freud) 112
metabolising-transformative function 2
metalanguage 9
metaphor, experiencing (inability) 62–63
metaphorical function 2
metaphorical thought, expression 64
metapsychological widening 1
metapsychology 5
"metapsychology of the third type"
    hypothesis 114
micro-expansions 111
micro-histories: expression 104–105;
    margins 105
micro-melody, discovery 37–38
micro-variations 111
middle age, dissociative crises 69
mien, changes 21
mind: concept, study 26; dissociated places
    34–36; nonexistence 26; psychosensory
    area, characteristics 5; sounding, mental
    capacity 72; symbolic-metaphorical
    function, access 62; theories 10–11
mirroring mechanisms 4
misunderstanding, initiation 53
mnemic traces 18
momentary impact, production 27
Momigliano, Luciana Nissim 70, 75
monadic subjectivities, uniting 92
Morpurgo, Enzo 72, 74, 89
Moses and Monotheism (Freud) 30
mother-child relationship, physical
    experience (working-through) 6
mother/child, social/emotional exchanges 8
mother-infant dyad 7–8
motility, usage 27
motor gesture 17
movement, power 57–58
"movement towards language" 109
"murmur of things" 22–23
muscular movements, analysis 21
musical listening 84
musical polyphony 38
"Music of What Happens, The" (Ogden) 39
mutism (result), deafness (impact) 89

narcissism, illness 91
narcissistic gratification 72
narcissistic-identity problems 75

narcissistic pathologies, increase 91
narrative humus, fostering 115
narratology 115
nascent movements, determination 6
Nebenmensch (nearest human being)
    (Freud) 56
Negation (Freud) 18
negative: aspects 15–16, 31; functions
    17–18; listening 15–20; understanding
    17, 18
negative capability 51
negative hallucination 16
negative traces: revealing, analytic listening
    (usage) 16; shape 11
negativisation 16
negativity 108
negatory narcissistic deals, construction 91
nervous illness, symptoms 112
never-alphabetised experiences,
    integration 83
"new clinical practices" (evidence) 104
new object, analyst (equivalence) 116
Night (Wiesel) 91
nighttime fantasy, dream disguise 15
noise: background noise 55; fright 49
non-linear dynamic systems 8
non-relationship, relationship (paradox) 35
non-represented, origin 12–15
non-specialists, shared culture 91–92
non-subjectivated object, identification 53
non-verbal communication: mediator 61;
    usage 83–84
non-verbal logics 8
non-verbal mental categories, usage 7
nostalgia, lullaby 86
not-known, encounter 77
not-me: me, distinction (achievement)
    56; potential 3; reality, cold
    extraneousness 95
not-other-than himself 53

object: awareness 53–54; entanglement
    36; experience 54; form, giving 52–55;
    iconic use 59; listening, presence
    (forms) 75–78; not-other-than himself
    53; presence, quality (revealing) 29;
    recognition/valuation 54; response 78;
    symbolising function 109–110
object-representation 51
object-subject: conceptualisation 5;
    presence 76
oedipal representation 104

Oedipus complex 92
omnipotent-omniscient expansion 36
"On Psychotherapy" (Freud) 40
"On the Music of Thought" (Seiden) 81
open sesame 82–83, 85
other (Other): annihilating/persecutory
    presence 63; experiencing, primordial
    representations 58; intrusion 62;
    presence 76; recognition 92; self-harm/
    harm 69
otherness, metabolising 96
other-than-oneself, generative
    encounters 70
other-than-self: communication, skin
    (psychic function) 95–97; contact 95;
    physical/emotional contact, desire 69;
    visual field perception 95
Outline of Psychoanalysis (Freud) 24

pacifiers 90
Pagnoni, Adriana 74
pain, alleviation 54
painting, "putting on" 117
panic attacks, generation 33
para-excitation (Skin-Ego function) 96
parental dependency, relationship
    (development) 52
parents, rivalry 92
Parsons, Michael 73
partner, motivations 49
passifiers 90
passionate speech 19
passionate speech (Fusini) 3
passiveness, involvement 11
past experiences, symmetries/resonances 32
pathogenic relationships, reproduction 58
pathos/logos, constant conjunction
    (maintenance) 117
patient(s): actions, availability 19;
    feelings, intensity 21; hearing, destiny
    (interpretation) 76; heterogenous
    patients, recalling 48–49; information,
    supply 9; internal narrator, encounter
    116–117; interpretation, implementation
    111; life-story production, plastic
    clarity 11; meaning, abstraction 73;
    psychic movement, creation 9; repressed
    material, impact 31; shared repetition
    in action 32; subjectivity, analyst-object
    physical presence (impact) 75;
    suffering, welcoming 72; unconscious,
    transmission 21

patient-analyst: affective/emotional communication 14; communication, unconscious reverberations 2–3
patrimony, value 78
peer relationship, bonding 72
perceiving (data functioning/gathering register) 5
perception: data derivation 19; identity, concept 58
perception-consciousness, conceptual binomial (openness) 11
perceptual environment, diectic use 59
perceptual experiences 5
personal psychic world, construction 81
perspectives (creation), interpretation (usage) 86
per via di levare 72, 111
per via di porre 72
philia, potency/discussion 92
phobia, processes 69–70
phobic avoidance 15
phonatory apparatus, evolution 59
physical aliveness 26
physical contact, desire 69
physical experience, working-through 6
physical malaise 32
physical state, interchange 6–7
physiological homeostasis, perturbation 57–58
physiological impression, engagement 3
physiological negative capability 16
Pillars of Hercules, psychoanalysis (relationship) 47
Pirandello, Luigi 35
plasticity 11
Playing and Reality (Winnicott) 15
poem, alphabet (presence) 3
poetry: academic commentaries 73; evocative word 93; metaphor 81; music, occurrence 81; strength 93
polymorphous associativity 19
polymorphous psyche 9
polymorphous psychic amalgams 107
polymorphous psychic materials, amalgam 13–14
polyphonic listening 108–109; indispensability 107
polyphonic polymorphous heteromorphous listening, associative modes (usage) 77–78
polysemic complexity 3
polysemy, construction (ability) 12

polytopia 12
porre 111
post-Bionian perspectives, changes 113
post-natal conscious, direction 24
posture, changes 21
pre-conscious representation 104
premature interpretations 79
pre-oedipal representation 104
pre-reflective mimetic openings 26
pre-representational affectivity 57
pre-representational phase 15
pre-representational sensoriality, impact 54
presence-absence-recognition, permutations 5
pre-symbolic, symbolic (caesura) 24
preverbal experience, sensory/sensual richness (sacrifice) 25
preverbal self, sense 25
preverbal, verbal (caesura) 24
primal incompleteness, condition 92
primal rule 92
primary defence: mechanisms 16; reactions 30
primary experiences, subjectivation process 69–70
primary maternal care 94
primary symbolisation, blockages (creation) 76–77
primitive agony, experience 15
primitive personal memory, usage 36
primordial representations 58
private self, vitality 7
projection (defensive strategy) 52
projective identification, concept 26
proleptic intuition 73
provisional constructions, usage 116–117
psyche: continuum 23; event, dialogue (complexity) 28; extension 26; invasion 55–56; knowledge 23; oscillation 36–37; unconscious, relationship 14
psyche-skin relationship 94
psyche-soma 11, 26; communication level 27; experience 87; levels, utilisation 27; work 59–61
psychic: composite structure 20–21; expression, heterogeneous forms (re-presentation) 21; formation 11
psychic action, configuration 18
psychical field, reproduction 59
psychic apparatus, theory 93–94
psychic, composite structure 20–21
psychic constipation, avoidance 56

psychic development, structuring 25
psychic dynamics, organising signs 15
psychic economy, analytic pair
    (implications) 15–20
psychic elaboration, context 23
psychic experience, fragmentation
    (saturating) 35
psychic expressions, origin 8
psychic figurability, building 48
psychic form(s): giving 56–57; usage 1–2
psychic function(s): disorganisation/
    destruction 14; libidinal recharging,
    Skin-Ego function 96; mental quality 7
psychic functioning 48; archaic
    levels, reaching 97; knowledge 71;
    understanding 20
psychic gesture, action 23–24
psychic humus: providing 65;
    vivification 105
psychic inscriptions, differentiation
    (absence) 104
psychic intensities 1, 27; evocation 39;
    handling 30–31; usage 79
psychic interweaving 39
psychic knowledge, impact 10
psychic life: engine 13; origin 29
psychic material: integrating, goal
    (communication) 9; procuring 3
psychic movement: creation 9;
    identification 38–39
psychic operation 9
psychic realities 18
"Psychic Reality and Social Rules"
    (Borutti) 92
psychic representation, conception 17
psychic retreat 34–35
psychic skin 93–97
psychic-soma, early trauma (imprint) 34
psychic structures, formation 10
psychic subject 6–7
psychic territories, advances 4
psychic traces 28–29
psychic work: associative psychic work
    39; ceaselessness 5; forms 19; material,
    gathering 9; occurrence 80; vicissitudes,
    comprehension 35
psychoanalysis: action theory, absence 19;
    aspects 103; assumption 114;
    auditory dimension 73–74; birth
    82–83; development 107; discipline,
    appearance 91; dynamic psychoanalysis
    92; foundation 89; metaphor 81; music,

occurrence 81; problems/questions
    113–117; social dimension, promotion
    89; word, power 83
psychoanalytic culture, cat's cradle 112
psychoanalytic encounter 1
psychoanalytic functioning 57;
    conception 26
psychoanalytic instrument, quality 47
psychoanalytic knowledge, capacity
    (widening) 70
psychoanalytic koinē, allusion 103
psychoanalytic listening:
    metapsychological boundaries,
    extension 37; paradigm,
    metapsychological widening 1
psychoanalytic object 1
psychoanalytic process, unfolding 88
psychoanalytic status 4
psychoanalytic thinking, extension 21–22
psychoanalytic treatment, boundaries
    (widening) 31
psycho-corporeal integration 87
psychological survival 36
psychoneurosis, repressed unconscious 14
psychophysical functioning, registers 12
psychosomatic disorders 34
psychosomatic disturbances, functioning
    modes (relationship) 97–98
psychosomatic envelope 94
psychosomatic existence, beginning 26
psychosomatic functioning 57
psychosomatic resonances 2–3

Quinodoz, Danielle 48

Racalbuto, Agostino 84
rage, externalisation 17
read language 25
reality: defining, internal analytic setting
    73; transformation 55–56
re-appropriation, conditions/modes/
    function 114
recipient, attention/imagination
    (directing) 59
reciprocity 92
recognition, emotion (revealing) 38
recollection: absence 30; dynamics 24
re-creation, processes 86
referential activity 81–82
reflective functioning, levels 34
registers, involvement 20
registration, multiple codes 27–28

regression, impact 77
relational function 59–60
relationship: being/existence, logics
    (knowledge) 14; re-experiencing 97;
    training basis 76–77
Remembering, Repeating, and
    Working-Through (Freud) 12
representation 56–57; drive, example
    61–64; network 30
representational functions, formation
    (reciprocity) 5
representational organ 61
representations in action 53, 64
"representations of something" 24
repressed representation 104
repression, secondary processes 9;
    theory 10
reproduction, repetition form 58–59
resonance (capability), internal forces
    (impact) 3
"respectful listening" 70
restarts 111
return journey, function 113–114
reverberation time 111
robotic functioning 62

Sand, George 38
satisfaction, experience 27
sculpture, "taking away" 11
secondary elaboration (communicable
    derivative) 80
secondary repression: dimension, impact
    21–22; theory 10
Seeking System, studies (distinction) 7
self (Self): container, firmness 96;
    dissociated aspects, research 14;
    experience, disruption 34; facing 50–52;
    functioning 36; impoverishment 69;
    integrity 95–96; not-self, differentiation
    53, 63; other-than-self (communication),
    skin (psychic function) 95–97;
    proprioception 94; representations 56;
    sense, formation 57–58; separate self
    94; unintegrated states, persistence 58;
    uniting, skin (psychic function) 93–95
self-awareness, damage 30
self-containment, activation 94
self-destruction (Skin-Ego function) 96
self-expression, forms 22
selfobject (Kohut) 29
self-other boundaries 53
semantic migrations 39

semiotic function 2
semiotic gestures 22–23
semiotic unconscious, capability 27
sensation, subject 4
sense: absence 54; generative potential 54
sensorimotor correlates 18
sensorimotoricity, data derivation 19
sensorimotor stage 51
sensory coming to be 6
sensory experience, translation 25
sensory stimuli, usage 6
separate self 94
sessions, number (increase) 51
sexual excitation (Skin-Ego function) 96
shared communicative context 60
shared intentionality 60
shared unconscious communication,
    psychic forms (usage) 1–2
sibling bond, example 90, 91–93
signification, context 23
silence 49; listening, connection 88–90;
    praise 111; voices 88; zones 90–91
"silencers" 90
silent openness 72
Skin-Ego: envelope 95–96; form, giving
    95; functions 96
skin, psychic function 93–97
socialisation, Searle formula
    (application) 60
sociality, link establishment (inability) 91
somatic parts/feelings/functions,
    imaginative elaboration 26
somatopsychic malfunctioning, effects
    (treatment) 97
"Something More" Than Interpretation,
    The (Boston Change Process Study
    Group) 28
sonic-musical dimension 107
space-time, creation 71
spatial metaphor, illustration 35
speaking, internal inspiration (link) 86
specific actions 27
speech: communication 59–61;
    intercorporeality 59–61; language 27;
    sensory-motor elements 25
"spit out" (metaphor) 17
split-off, research 14
splitting (defensive strategy) 52, 78
splitting-dissociation 16
stable instability, maintenance 53, 56
stand-by, eternal state 84–85
Stern, Daniel 6

"stories never told" 105
stories, poverty 62
Studies on Hysteria (Freud) 82
subject: becoming, sisyphean labour 74;
    enigmatic privacy, word (relationship)
    88; *in fieri,* presence (signalling)
    74; prehistory, foregrounding 105;
    unconscious creativity, object presence
    (constant dialogue) 29
subjectivated body-ego 57
subjectivated existence 74
subjectivation: possibility 75;
    process 16, 48
subjective appropriation: achievement 74;
    forms/permutations, rethinking 29
subjective experience, symbolic
    appropriation 108
subjective reappropriation 109, 115
subjective state, interchange 6–7
subjectivity 92, 115; acknowledgement,
    failure 54; construct 33; moments,
    attention 71–72
subject-object relationship, traumatic
    quality 36
submission, dynamic 16
sub-symbolic states 84
subtle interplay, understanding 20–21
suitable acts 27
Superego, introjection 112
superficial association 50–51
support (Skin-Ego function) 96
suspended attention 72
symbol formation, illusion (role) 12
symbolic function 2
symbolic-metaphorical function, access 62
symbolic orders, compatibility relations 12
symbolic, pre-symbolic (caesura) 24
symbolic representation (communicable
    derivative) 80
symbolic-representative function,
    reactivation 62
symbolic solutions, production 12
symbolic speaking 63
symbolic thought, expression 64
symbolic transformation 55–56
symbolisation 18, 109–110; approach 30;
    process 16, 104, 109; theme, reflections
    12–15
symbolising form, achievement 8
symbolising function, subject
    (relationship) 105
symbolising object, trace 109

"symbolism in time" 13
symbols, clearing 69–71
synchronisation, elements 19–20
synchrony, diachrony (contrast) 71

tactile sensory traces, registering (Skin-Ego
    function) 96
talking cure 61, 82–83
technique, refinement 48
Telescoping of Generations, The
    (Faimberg) 75
temporality (temporalities): creation 13;
    plurality, determination 11, 20–21
temporal short-circuit 96
tension, freedom 72
terza rima rhyme, usage 87
theoretical-clinical discursive strategy 109
therapeutic action 12
therapeutic position, matrix
    (embodiment) 72
therapists: analytic listening 72;
    role 97–98
therapy, payment 79
thing-representation 61
things: murmur 22–23; words, caesura 24
thinkability, conditions (pre-interpretative
    weaving) 110
thinking: concreteness 62–63; formal
    regression 77
thinking heart: encounter 74; search 84
thin-skinned psychic envelopes 15
Third Reich, secret code 90
thoughts: dream-thoughts, translation 80;
    existing, possibility 22; possibility,
    disorganising 55–56
"thought without language" 24–25
tonal modulations 111
tongues, confusion 29
*topographically significant mental
    representations,* construction 14
traces: mnemic traces 18; plurality,
    determination 11, 20–21; preservation,
    ability 24; psychic traces 28–29
transference(s) 48, 52, 104–108; displays
    9; distinctiveness 18; dynamic 16–17;
    extension 104–105; history, connection
    104–105; material, extension 105;
    relationship 52; transformative
    transference 105; triple translational
    transference 107; usage 12
transference-countertransference: dialogue
    1–2; relationship 49

transferential-countertransferential scenario 64–65
transferential intensity 79
transferential reawakenings, impact 16
transferential repetition, potentiality 16
transformation (cure): factors 110–112; process, heterogeneity 5; psychic work 5; risk 111; search 64
transformation *à deux* 19
transformative factors, change 110
transformative object, communicative link 1
transformative transference 105
transgenerational hierarchy 92
transitionality 109
transitional object: construction 13; infant usage 13; meaninglessness 13
trans-lation 105
transpersonal dreaming situation, impact 113
transpersonal interchanges 115
trans-psychic intrusion 111
trauma, imprint 34
traumatic dimensions, reflections 28–31
traumatic experiences, impact 34
traumatic factor, interrogation 15–16
traumatic memory, enactments 61
traumatic traces 16
Traumdeutung (Freud) 58
treatment, capacity 70
triple translational transference 107
"true psychoanalytic interpretation," boundaries 110
Turgenev, Ivan 38
Turing, Alan 90
Two Principles of Mental Functioning (Freud) 10–11

unconscious: assumptions (Freud) 40; contents, emergence 69–70; dialogue 78; expression, field (opening) 10; Freud formulation 14; heterogeneous emergences, listening 1; non-linguistic nature, revelation 26; speaking, ability 9
unconscious aspects, creative/integrating activity (link) 86
unconscious communication(s) 20, 61; concept 26; consideration 21; occurrence 70
unconscious cooperation 19
unconscious creativity, object presence (constant dialogue) 29

unconscious currents, catching 9–12
unconscious dialects, usage 24
unconscious intersubjective construction, forms (listening) 20–22
unconscious meanings, emotional schemata (transcription) 33
unconsciousness: communication 21; embodied unconsciousness 47
unconscious object, production/ investigation 73
unconscious organisation 20
unconscious polytopia 12
unconscious psychic life, existence 78
unconscious reception, configurations 10
unconscious social processes 78
unconscious work 86
unconscious world, subjectivation 77
understanding: approach 2; language, impact 2
unformulated thoughts, approach 22
uniform experience, ingredients (accentuation) 25
unknown unconscious space, usage 78
unthought future 105
urgency, feeling (inclusion) 50
utterances, emphasis 10

Valduga, Partrizia 87–88
verbal clarity 49
verbal communication, usage 83–84
verbal expressions, translation 18
verbal language 11
verbal, preverbal (caesura) 24
verbal relatedness domain 25
verbal relations 28
verbal scribbling 39
verbal thinking, impact 8
Verneinung (denial), concept 18
Verwerfung (Freud concept) 34
Vigne, Pier Delle (suicide) 87
viscera, movement (elements) 20
vital affective dynamic 20
voice: ignoring 90; tones, sequence (revealing) 10
"voices of the silence" 88
vulnerability, reminding 97

Wiesel, Elie 91
Wittgenstein, Ludwig 59
wo Es war (subjective experience) 108
women, stereotyped descriptions 51

wordplay, capacity (usage) 39
word-representations, hallucinatory
    potential 77
words: affect 82; communication,
    centrality 84; condensation 80–82;
    condensed words, listening 80; envelope
    93–97; fullness 88; immersion 97–98;
    importance 86; intensities 78–79;
    island-words, sonic material 73–75;
    listening, openings 69; "magic" word,
    power 82–88; orchestration, absence 81;
    power 83–85; representation,
    absence 31–34; uttering 25
"work as a double" 11, 21
working-through 32
wounding, absence 72
written language 25

You-I direction 60
youthful breakdown 69

zones of silence 90–91